INTERNATIONAL COMPARATIVE STUDY OF COMMUNITY NURSING

International Comparative Study of Community Nursing

ROBERT A. VERHEIJ
ADA KERKSTRA
Netherlands Institute of Primary Health Care (NIVEL)

Avebury

Aldershot · Brookfield USA · Hong Kong · Singapore · Sydney

Published by
Avebury
Ashgate Publishing Limited
Gower House
Croft Road
Aldershot
Hants GU 11 3 HR
England

Ashgate Publishing Company
Old Post Road
Brookfield
Vermont 05036
USA

A CIP catalogue record for this book is available from the British Library and the US Library of Congress

Typeset by
M.A.M. van der Meulen-Kimmelaar
NIVEL - Utrecht - The Netherlands

ISBN 1 85628 415 8

Printed and Bound in Great Britain by
Athenaeum Press Ltd., Newcastle upon Tyne.

Contents

Preface

This book gives a description and comparison of the organization, funding and functioning of community nursing organizations in Belgium, Canada, Finland, France, Germany, the Netherlands, Norway, the United Kingdom and the United States.

The research project was funded by the Dutch Ministry of Welfare, Health and Cultural Affairs and conducted by the Netherlands Institute of Primary Health Care (NIVEL).

The authors would like to express their gratitude to all those who have participated in the study.

Furthermore, we thankfully acknowledge the help of Mrs M. de Jong (Vereniging voor Verpleegkundigen en Verzorgenden in de Maatschappelijke gezondheidszorg [Dutch Association of Nurses]), Mr R. Laagewaard (Dutch Ministry of Welfare, Health and Cultural Affairs, department of general health care and professions), Mrs F.J. Mensink (Department of nursing Science, Hogeschool Midden Nederland) and Mrs R. van Vliet (Health Inspectorate), members of the counselling committee.

We would like to thank Mrs M. van der Meulen for the wordprocessing and lay-out, and Mr P. van der Heijden for his kind help writing some paragraphs.

Robert Verheij
Ada Kerkstra

Introduction

The purpose of this study is to provide information about the organization, functioning and funding of community nursing in various industrialized countries. This information should serve as a background for future develop ments concerning community nursing in the Netherlands. In other words, we will try to learn from the experience of other countries: about their problems and their attempts to solve these problems.

This is not easy, and we will easily be tempted to adopt solutions in the Netherlands that have proved to work in other countries, without paying enough attention to the unique factors in those other countries. Each country has its own historical background, each country has its own way of organizing health care in general, each country has its own geographical features.

This, however, should not prevent us from looking at those other countries, since there are indeed a lot of common features. All industrialized countries, for instance, are confronted with an ageing population. In most countries the proportion of elderly is higher than in the Netherlands. All industrialized countries are trying to limit the costs of health care and many countries do this by trying to substitute home care for hospital care and shortening the average length of stay in hospital. It will be interesting to see how other countries cope with the growing demand for home care, which is caused by these developments. It will, furthermore, be interesting to compare the organization of home care elsewhere with the organizational changes in home care that are being proposed in the Netherlands.

Furthermore, with the arrival of the magical year 1993 and the free move- ment of people within Europe connected with it, it may be useful to know what an immigrant nurse from for instance France has been doing in her mother country. What her responsibilities have been and how she has been trained.

Background and purpose of the study

Large organizational changes are being carried out in the Dutch health care system. They all affect the organization of home care directly or indirectly. Additionally, the population is ageing, causing a greater need for home care. Below we will give a short description of the current issues.

Elderly population Three factors cause a growing proportion of elderly in the Dutch population.

First of all, less children are being born, which results in an increasing proportion of elderly in the total population.

Second, the post-war baby boom generation is rapidly becoming old, which will cause a relative increase in the elderly population within 15 to 25 years.

Third, developments in medical science and higher standards of living are causing life expectancy to increase. The elderly are going to live much longer than they used to 30 years ago.

Government policy Since it was confronted with the rising costs of health care a few decades ago, the government has proposed several measures to reduce these costs.

Home care is considered cheaper than hospital care. So, since the nineteen seventies, the government has planned to substitute home care for hospital care, aided by the increasing technological options enabling the provision of care at home that could previously only be delivered in hospitals. This policy can be considered successful, as the average length of stay in hospital has dropped from 12.7 days in 1982 to 11.8 in 1986 (CBS 1991). The Netherlands is not the only country that has adopted this policy: 'The one public policy principle common to all twelve EC countries (..) is that the elderly should stay in their own homes for as long as possible (Nijkamp et al., 1991).

Another measure that is generally considered to reduce the costs, is the introduction of competition between health care providers. Competition will be introduced in the health care system, within the next 5 years. Nor is the Netherlands alone in this respect: "Many other countries are beginning to encourage private sector activity in elderly care" (Nijkamp et al., 1991).

Organization of home care Until 1989, home help services and community nursing services, which are the most important providers of home care in the Netherlands, each had their own organization. Although this did not mean that there was no co-ordination and co-operation between the two organizations, it was still considered to be more efficient if both types of services were delivered by the same organization. In 1990 the umbrella organizations for home help services and community nursing services merged.

In the coming years the lower levels, at which the care is delivered, will merge too. This will have consequences for the division of tasks and responsibilities between home helps and nurses with a lower level of expertise. Furthermore, methods of assessment of patient need will have to be adapted to the new situation and be combined for home help and nursing care.

The new situation will also contribute to the debate as to whether community nurses should work as generalists or specialists.

Preventive activities will suffer from the increasing curative workload. The question is whether community nurses can continue to continue to work both in child health care and home care for elderly. Furthermore, because of epidemiological changes, substitution of home care for hospital care and the increasing use of the options of technically advanced medical treatment at home the nature and complexity of the demand for home care is changing. Consequently, an increasing need is felt for a more specialized approach to community nursing.

Finally, there is a (threatening) shortage of community nurses. According to the Commission Werner (1991) there is a feeling of dissatisfaction among community nurses. Heavy workload, lack of appreciation, less well-defined tasks and responsibilities and lack of autonomy are mentioned as reasons for this dissatisfaction.

The reason for this study is that we believe that the issues described above are not unique for the Dutch situation and that it may be useful to look at other countries.

In the study we will try to answer the following questions for each country:

1   How is community nursing organized?
2   How is community nursing funded?
3   What levels of expertise are there among nurses?
4   What specializations are there among nurses?
5   What arrangements are there concerning the division of tasks and responsibilities between nurses?
6   How is the assessment carried out?
7   How do organizations co-operate with other care providers (home help services, general practitioners and hospitals)?
8   What problems are there in the provision of community nursing care?

Method

Selection of countries   An initial limitation was made by selecting the 24 countries that take part in the Organization of Economic Cooperation and Development (OECD). However, even between these 24 countries, there are large differences in Gross Domestic Products (GDP), and consequently in the quantity of resources available to health care. We decided to take only the richest countries into account, leaving out Italy, Turkey, Portugal, Greece,

3

Spain and Ireland. Iceland and Luxembourg were excluded because of their small population.

From among the remaining countries, Canada, the United States, Norway, Finland, Great-Britain, (the Federal Republic of) Germany, Belgium, France and the Netherlands were selected.

This group was chosen, first, because it included countries with a strict division between primary and secondary care in terms of accessability, as well as countries in which such a division does not obtain. Great Britain, Finland and the Netherlands are representatives of the first category (secondary care requires a referral by a GP), France, Germany, Belgium, Canada and the United States of the second (no referral needed), while Norway belongs to both (free access to secondary care in Oslo and referral system in the rest of the country).

Second, in the Netherlands most nurses work as generalists, while in the other countries various distinctions are made between preventive care and curative care in educational programs as well as in the organization of community nursing care.

Third, there are countries with special features which can be of interest in the Dutch situation. The United States for example has a large profit-making sector in community nursing, in France the organization of community nursing is still in an early stage of development, in Germany home help services are often part of the same organization as community nursing services.

Desk research   The literature in the files of NIVEL, the University of Utrecht, and the Central Bureau of Statistics has been investigated. Additionally, three international databases were consulted: Cinahl, Medline and Excerpta Medica. The key words used were: community nursing, home health nursing, home care, Gemeindekrankenpflege, Bezirkskrankenpflege, Sozialstationen and wijkverpleging, all in combination with the nine selected countries.

Experts   Our aim was to find experts on community nursing in each country and to ask them to complete a questionnaire. Preference was given to people engaged in research into community nursing, hoping they would be able to provide a national overview for their country.

The search for experts in each country took place using:
-    personal contacts established during the International Conference on Community Nursing organized by NIVEL in 1989;
-    contacts of the Regional Office of the World Health Organization in Copenhagen;
-    contacts through the European Association of Organizations for Home Care and Help at Home;

-	contacts of the Dutch National Association for Home Care.
From these contacts a list of potential participants resulted. These were asked to participate in the study. If they were unable to participate they were asked whether they knew other persons who could be considered experts on community nursing and who would possibly be willing to participate.

In the USA and France and to some extent Canada the large variety of organizations inhibited a national overview. In these countries the questionnaires were therefore sent to organizations that were indicated by other national experts on the basis of their own personal contacts with these organizations.

Questionnaire In October and November 1990 a comprehensive questionnaire was developed in the English language and mailed in December.

In the questionnaire community nursing organizations were defined as follows:

Type of care
Organizations included in this study may deliver rehabilitative, supportive, promotive or preventive care, including medical technical care. Organizations specializing in one of these types of care should also be taken into account.

Location
This care will have to be delivered in the 'community'. In practice this means that most of the care is delivered to non-institutionalized people, living in their own homes. It is, however, possible that *some* of the care may also delivered to institutionalized people.

Funding
Organizations may be either for-profit or not-for-profit.

Specialization
Organizations may specialize in certain types of care or certain groups in the population. Organizations specializing in the following are excluded: psychiatric care; midwifery; school health nursing and occupational nursing.

Personnel
The organization must employ nurses (in the widest sense of the word). The personnel may include physicians and/or home help aides, though this is not necessary.

5

Importance
The organization will have to be of importance in the sense that it serves a considerable part of the population. The meaning of the word 'considerable' will have to be determined by the respondent him/herself.

Respondents were asked to compose a list of organizations to which the above definition applied and to make a selection of organizations for which they were able to complete the questionnaire.

After having made a selection of organizations to which the answers would apply respondents were asked about the following topics:
- Organizational structure
- Government regulations
- History of the organization
- Funding of the organization and payment of nurses
- Patient populations, size and composition
- Types of care delivered to these populations; proportion of working time spent on selected activities
- Types of personnel; who they are, what they do, how many there are
- Stages in nursing; initiators of first contact, use of assessment guides
- Co-operation with other care providers
- Problems; activities subject to under-performance; shortages and their reasons.

Some questions were preceded by short a introduction that was meant to show the rationale behind each question. In addition, the questionnaire was answered by the authors for the Dutch situation in advance and these answers were enclosed in the questionnaire.

Response In December 1990 a total number of 32 questionnaires was mailed. The number of questionnaires mailed to each country was dependent on the presumed complexity of the organization of community nursing. After two months a reminder was sent to those who had not yet answered. A total number of 23 questionnaires were completed (Table I). Part of the non-response may be attributed to problems with the language (mainly in France) and another part to the comprehensiveness and time consuming nature of the questionnaire.

A list of respondents to the questionnaire is provided in Appendix 1.

Table I
Number of questionnaires mailed, response and number of reviewers by country

	no. of questionnaires mailed	no. of respondents	no. of reviewers
Belgium	4	3	2
Canada	3	2	1
England	3	3	3
Finland	2	1	1
France	8	3	1
Germany	5	5	2
Netherlands	-	-	-
Norway	2	2	2
USA	5	4	1
total	32	23	13

Visits In addition to the questionnaire and desk research, four countries were visited by one of the authors in February and April 1991. During these visits the actual practice of community nursing was observed for 1 or 2 days and the experts in these countries were personally consulted. The four countries were Finland, England, France and Germany. The organizations that were visited were chosen by (one of) the experts in each country. A list of organizations that were visited is provided in Appendix 2.

Reviewing Draft chapters on each country were written based on information from the literature, questionnaires and visits. These chapters were consequently reviewed to check them for too much biased information. As a rule the experts who responded to the questionnaire were also asked to review the text, in this way partly checking each other's information.

Finland forms a special case. Here the one respondent consulted others on her own.

In the USA and France with their large variety of organizations it was considered better to ask other people to review the text, people who were assumed to have a somewhat broader view of community nursing in their country than the respondents to the questionnaire.

Contents of the study

The following chapters are concerned with a description of community nursing in the selected countries. Before coming down to community nursing itself, however, it is necessary to become aware of the national context in which community nursing operates.

Consequently, the description of each country starts with some information about the health care system. This is done in two parts: the first describing relevant features of the population; the second giving a short introduction to the providers of health care, their role and number, and giving information about the funding of health care.

The description of characteristics of the health care system is followed by a descriptive analysis of community nursing in each country. The results from the questionnaire will be presented here, supplemented by literature. In some countries there is more than one organization concerned with community nursing as we define it. We have tried to include the most important organizations in these countries, resulting in a rather cursory description of separate organizations in France, Canada and the USA. In some countries it appeared only to be possible to discuss the provision of curative (elderly-) care. Table II gives the main sources of data in the various chapters and states whether preventive care was included or not.

Chapter 10 will be concerned with cross national comparison. In this chapter we shall try to compare the most important features of community nursing in each country and draw some general conclusions.

For reasons of brevity nurses are referred to as 'she', in spite of the fact that a growing number of men enter the nursing profession nowadays.

Table II
Main sources of data for country descriptions and whether the focus is on curative of preventive care or both

	Sources	Focus
Belgium	Three organizations: White-Yellow Cross; Solidarity for the Family; Child and Family	curative + preventive
Canada	Victorian Order of Nurses in Ontario St. John's District Health Unit, New Foundland	curative + preventive
Finland	General overview	curative + preventive
France	Two organizations for home care	curative
Germany	National overview Sozialstationen	curative
Netherlands	General overview Cross Associations	curative + preventive
Norway	General overview	curative + preventive
UK	District Nursing; Health Visiting; Community Psychiatric Nursing in England	curative + preventive
USA	Two Visiting Nurse Associations	curative

References

CBS. (1991), *Statistical Yearbook of the Netherlands,* Central Bureau of Statistics, 's-Gravenhage.

Commissie Werner (Commissie positiebepaling beroep van verpleegkundige en verzorgende) (1991), *In hoger beroep. Perspectief voor de verplegende en verzorgende beroepen* [Perspectives for nursing and caring personnel], Ministerie van WVC, Rijswijk.

Nijkamp, P., J. Pacolet, H. Spinnewyn, A. Vollering, C. Wilderom, S. Winters (1991), *Services for the elderly in Europe; A cross-national comparative study,* Commission for the European Communities, Leuven.

1 Community nursing in Belgium

The setting [1]

Population [2]

* total population (1987)   9,9 million
* % over 65 (1988)   14,3
* % over 65 (2000, projected)   14,7
* % over 65 (2010, projected)   15,9
* % over 65 (2020, projected)   17,7
* % under 15 (1988)   18,3
* life expectancy at birth (years) (1982/83)   70,5 (men)
                                                            77,2 (women)
* live births per 1000 inhabitants (1988)   11,8
* population density per sq. kilometre (1987)   325
* population groups: Belgium is a trilingual country, with Dutch being spoken in the north and French in the south and a small German speaking minority in the east. There has been some immigration from Mediterranean countries during the sixties, seventies and eighties. In addition, there are some cultural minorities from former Belgian colonies in Africa.

Health care system [3]

Introduction   Belgium is a constitutional monarchy. The country is divided between Flemings, the Dutch-speaking community and Walloons, the French-speaking community. Separate community governments exists for Brussels and the German speaking "Ostkanton".

To some extent Belgium is a federal state, with four parts: Flanders, the Walloon provinces, Brussels and the Ostkanton. Extensive decision-making power is delegated to these Communities.

Health insurance The compulsory health care costs and disability insurance covers ninety-nine percent of the population. Two insurance schemes exist: the general scheme for all employees, their dependents and pensioners, and the independent scheme for the self-employed. The independent scheme is designed to insure only hospital admissions, while the coverage of the general scheme is broader.

The health insurance system is based on the principle of reimbursement. The patient pays the doctor and hands the bill in at his local health insurance office, except for hospital bills which are usually directly paid by the health insurance fund to the hospitals.

Another characteristic of the health insurance system is the existence of co-payments (which may be up to 25% for ambulatory care). Not all health service charges are reimbursed. Disabled persons, widows, pensioners and orphans are almost completely exempted from these co-payments ('Ticket Moderateur'). The amount of co-payment is determined by the Community Government. The health insurance fund offer additional insurance for co-payments, on a voluntary basis.

The statutory insurance scheme is operated by the private, autonomous decentralized Health Insurance Funds. The local health insurance funds are united in six national organizations with differing religious, political, and trade union affiliations, which are in turn supervised by the National Sickness and Disability Fund (RIZIV). The communities (Flanders, Walloon, Brussels and the Ostkanton) are responsible for setting the minimal standards for health care provision, management of social services, care for the aged, health education and home-care. At the national level, there are tasks in health insurance, hospital legislation, professional education and quality of care in general.

Table 1.1
Total and public expenditure on health in Belgium (percent of GDP)

year	total expend. % GDP	public. expend. % GDP
1980	6.69	5.46
1981	7.17	5.77
1982	7.20	5.76
1983	7.38	5.66
1984	7.35	5.63
1985	7.37	5.67
1986	7.36	5.66
1987	7.45	5.73

Source: Program ECO-SANTE by BASYS/CREDES

Ambulatory care   Medical care outside the hospitals is provided by the numerous GPs as well as by private specialists both operating from their surgeries on a solo-practice basis. Group practices do exist but are still a minority. There is no sharp division of tasks between GPs and ambulatory specialists. Belgians are free to consult any physician inside or outside hospitals without referral. Nevertheless there may be referrals. For instance from a GP to an ambulatory or hospital-based specialist or unspecified to an outpatient department. The same goes for the ambulatory specialist. There is a free doctor choice for every consultation. General Practitioners are paid on a fee for service basis.

The total number of physicians in 1990 was about 35,000 of which some 16,000 GPs and some 19,000 specialists [4]. Belgium had 3,5 physicians per 1000 inhabitants. This is very high compared to other European countries (2,8 in Germany, 1,37 in Great Britain and 2,35 in the Netherlands in 1987) (Koster et al., 1991).

Institutional care   The patient has complete freedom of choice with regard to the institution. These institutions either belong to the public or to the private sector. All general hospitals run outpatient departments. Emergency cases are sent to public or private hospitals that run an emergency department.

Mean length of stay in somatic hospitals in days (1980) (OECD, 1987): 13.5

Table 1.2
Inpatient medical care beds and personnel per bed

years	beds total	beds per 1000	personnel per bed
1980	91889	9.3	1.04
1981	92436	9.4	1.06
1982	92686	9.4	1.10
1983	92138	9.3	1.12
1984	91638	9.3	1.13
1985	90790	9.2	1.15
1986	89589	9.1	1.21
1987	88554	9.0	1.25

Source: Program ECO-SANTE by BASYS/CREDES

Community nursing

Leaving aside a small German speaking minority and Brussels, Belgium is a bilingual, federalized country and many activities are organized either for Flanders or the Walloon provinces. This is partly true for community nursing also. Accordingly, before discussing community nursing in Belgium we have to stress the fact that we are primarily concerned with Flanders. In the following sections we will concentrate on the most important providers of community nursing care: the 'Wit-Gele Kruis' (White-Yellow Cross) providing mainly curative care in both Flanders and the Walloon provinces and 'Kind en Gezin' (Child and Family), the only provider of child health care in Flanders. In addition, attention will be paid to a Flemish organization that combines community nursing services with home help and other services: Solidariteit voor het Gezin (Solidarity for the Family). This organization provides almost the same service as the White-Yellow Cross but the organizations do not compete.

In addition to organized community nursing care there are a substantial number of independent nurses "Liberales" who are self-employed.

History

White-Yellow Cross An important element of Belgian community nursing originated in religious orders. Another developed from health insurance funds though some of the organizations founded by health insurance funds and religious organizations still exist, the most important organization nowadays is the White-Yellow Cross, a federation of cross organizations founded in 1936. One of the most important historical events was the coming into force in 1963 of a 'national committee of agreement' (Voskuilen, 1991), in which health insurance funds and nurses negotiate national agreements on tariffs in nursing.

Solidarity for the Family Solidarity for the family came into existence in 1977. The organization started as a home help service in East Flanders. In 1979 the services were extended with community nursing, creating one of the first organizations that offer integrated home care, responding to a great need for professional nursing and hygienic care at home. In the same year a house-keeping service was added. In the following years a handyman service (1981), pedicure (1980), hairdresser (1984), nursing for mother and child (1985), meals on wheels (1986) and cultural, occupational therapy and educational centers were started.

Recent initiatives concern in-service training for home helpers and co-ope-ration initiatives (recognized as such by the Flemish government).

Child and Family The organization of preventive care for children developed from the 'National Child Welfare Agency' (Nationaal Werk voor Kinderwel-zijn, NWK), which was founded after an experiment with child care in the broadest sense of the word (including for instance the provision of milk at schools) during the first world war. Up until 1984 the NWK organized mother and child (health) care, child day care centres and residential care centres for mothers and children. This usually was done by supporting (existing) local initiatives rather than founding new local organizations (Vandenberghe, 1984).

In 1984, it was decided that child care should no longer be a national responsibility. Instead, two organizations were founded, one of which would take care of the French speaking community in southern Belgium and one to take care of the Dutch speaking community in the north. In Flanders, the service Child and Family was founded (Vandenberghe, 1984).

Although formally founded in 1984, it was not until 1987 that Child and Family actually commenced its work (Commissariat-General for International Co-operation - Flemish Community, 1990).

Organization and funding

Organization White-Yellow Cross The White-Yellow Cross is the most important provider of curative home care in Belgium.

Figure 2.1 shows the structure of the organization of the White-Yellow Cross.

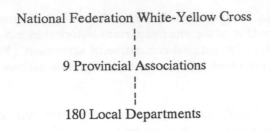

National Federation White-Yellow Cross

9 Provincial Associations

180 Local Departments

Figure 2.1 Structure of the organization of the White-Yellow Cross

Source: Wit-Gele Kruis van België, 1990

At the local level, each department employs 20 to 40 nurses, lead by a head nurse. Nurses usually work in a team, but within a team, each nurse takes care of her own specific area.

The provincial associations support and control the local departments and determine the number of nurses at the local level. The National Federation in turn supports the provincial associations, develops policy in co-operation with the provincial associations and represents these in contacts with ministries, social associations and professional organizations (Source: questionnaire).

Specialist knowledge on nursing is available at the national level in the form of some supporting committees for example on cancer. In 1990 a national technical committee of the White-Yellow Cross provided a syllabus on prevention of back pain. At the provincial level there are similar associations and at the local level there may be nurses who have taken specialist courses in back pain or diabetics, for instance. In 1989 the White-Yellow Cross organized practice oriented courses on palliative care and management at the local as well as provincial levels (Wit-Gele Kruis van België, 1990).

The White-Yellow Cross can be reached 24 hours a day and care can be delivered in the evenings, nights and weekends if necessary.

The Solidarity for the Family Organization Within the organization there are two heads of services: one for home help and housekeeping services (including meals on wheels and handyman services) and one for nursing services (including pedicure and hairdressing). The organization is further divided into regions. The nursing service regions are further divided into sectors for a number of which a social nurse (see below) is responsible. The social nurse is responsible for an average of about 20 nurses. A total number of 120 nurses is employed by Solidarity.

Nursing services can be reached by telephone 24 hours a day. Most other services only during office hours.

Child and Family Organization Child and Family is organized as follows. A board of governors is advised by the Provincial Committees and the Interdisciplinary Advice Committee. The latter sometimes establishes special committees that provide advice on particular issues such as antenatal care, day nurseries etc. (Commissariaat-Generaal voor de Internationale Samenwerking, 1990).

Furthermore, at the national level there are departments of General Services Administrative Affairs, Quality Control (covering quality supervision, in-service training and information), Child Care Services (including day care, maternity care, preventive child care and special residential care) and In House Care Services (services organized by own nursing staff) (Commissariaat-Generaal voor de Internationale Samenwerking, 1990).

A distinction is made between in-house and outside care services (Commissariaat-Generaal voor de Internationale Samenwerking, 1990), the first referring to all activities for which Child and Family carries full responsibility and which are initiated by Child and Family itself, the second referring to activities and services organized by private initiative.
In practice 'in-house' care refers to
- care during pregnancy
- post-natal care
- one 'child and family' residential care centre near Brussels, in addition to those already supported by private initiative.
- adoption
'Outside' care facilities
- various facilities for child day care
- facilities for cases of child abuse and neglect
Care during pregnancy and post-natal care is delivered by social nurses (sociaal verpleegkundigen) in the community. These nurses visit women during pregnancy and after childbirth, assist physicians in child health centres (consultatiebureaus voor het jonge kind) and hold information sessions. Social nurses hold a permanent appointment with Child and Family, while general practitioners, pediatricians and gynecologists with whom they cooperate (see below) are paid on a fee for service basis. The nurses work on a solo basis, each being assigned to a specific geographical area.

At all levels nurses can consult others for specialist information. At the local level the practitioner in the 'consultatiebureau' (child health clinic), with whom the nurses co-operate can be consulted; at the provincial level there are medical advisors (pediatricians and gynecologists) and social nurses specialized in diabetics can be consulted; at the national level dieticians.

Funding White-Yellow Cross Health insurance funds are the most important financiers of the White-Yellow Cross (Table 1.3).

17

Table 1.3
Sources of income of the White-Yellow Cross

public insurance companies (health insurance funds)	93.7
patient's membership fees	3.5
other	2.8

Source: questionnaire

Besides the health insurance funds, other sources of income are patient fees and yearly membership fees, which vary between BF 500 and 1000 per family (Voskuilen, 1991). In most cases the patient fees do not have to be paid. A very small minority are not insured against 'small risks', however, and have to pay the full costs. Widows, handicapped and pensioners are exempted from this by law (Rijksinstituut voor ziekte- en invaliditeitsverzekering, 1990).

Furthermore, there are government subsidies for personnel and co-operation initiatives. Government subsidies for nursing personnel are only paid if the personnel is part of a team of at least 5 full-time equivalents. Co-operation initiatives are subsidized on the condition that GPs taking a part in them, teams of nurses, home help services, social services as well as three representatives of other disciplines. Furthermore, the initiative has to cover a population of at least 25,000 (Wauters, 1991). The regulations on government subsidies are different in the Walloon community.

Reimbursement by health insurance funds takes place on a fee-for-service basis. Until 1989 each nursing activity had its own price but this system changed partially into reimbursement per day of care for (very) dependent patients according to patient physical dependency profiles. The level of dependency is measured using a scale developed by Katz et al. (1963) to assess physical condition. In addition, a scale developed by Van Loon and Geys (1990) for psychic dependency and a scale assessing the living conditions of the patient are used to facilitate the assessment of need.

There are three patient categories:
- less dependent patients, with fee-for-service reimbursement according to a 'nomenclature', which only contains technical nursing procedures (no preventive activities).
- moderately dependent patients with low reimbursement per day of care.
- highly dependent patients with high reimbursement per day of care.

According to Van Loon, in a Belgian newspaper (De Standaard, 26 March 1991) the two last categories account for only 20 to 25% of the total number of patients, leaving the majority of patients still being reimbursed according to the 'nomenclature'.

This new system came into force only very recently (April 1, 1991) and it is not yet possible to say how it functions and if people are content with it.

Nurses working for organizations like the White-Yellow Cross are paid a monthly salary by the provincial associations that may vary between 39.602 BF (brevetted nurses) and 42.929 BF (graduated nurses) (Voskuilen, 1991).

Independent nurses are paid directly, à l'acte by the health insurance funds or they have a contract with some organization and will be paid by this organization. It has to be noted here that the National Federation of the Wit-Gele Kruis does not have direct influence on tariffs and budget-planning. These are determined by the association of health insurance funds (Rijksinstituut voor Ziekte- en Invaliditeitsverzekering, RIZIV) and professional nursing organizations (Voskuilen, 1991).

Funding Solidarity for the Family The nursing service of Solidarity is funded the same way as the White-Yellow Cross. The home help service requires a patient fee dependent on income with a minimum of BF 19 per hour.

Funding Child and Family Table 1.4 clearly shows that government subsidies are the most important source of income for Child and Family.

Table 1.4
Sources of income Child and Family in 1989

government subsidies	78.7%
parent contributions	20.8%
other	0.5%

Source: Kind en Gezin, 1990

Parent contributions are only paid for child day care facilities. The rest of the services provided by Child and Family is free of charge.

Types of community nurses and manpower

Education There are three training programs in nursing in Belgium (Schepers and Nys, 1985), representing three levels of expertise
1   graduate nurse (gegradueerd verpleegkundige): Two year basic training, followed by one year specialization in hospital nursing, psychiatric nursing or paediatric nurse. Specialization into social nursing or midwifery takes two years instead of one.
2   brevetted nurse (gebrevetteerd verpleegster): Three year training.
3   brevetted hospital assistant (gebrevetteerd ziekenhuisassistente). Two year education.

The program for graduated nurses and brevetted nurses are the same length. However, the program for brevetted nurses places more emphasis on the practical part of the job, and admission requirements are less strict. There is also a university program in nursing.

Manpower White-Yellow Cross Table 1.5 gives the various types of personnel employed by the White-Yellow Cross. The table clearly shows the growth of the number of personnel. The number of nurses shows an increase of about 70% between 1985 and 1990.

The table also shows a relatively high proportion of second (brevetted) level nurses. For each graduate nurse there is 1.5 brevetted nurse. Only a very small proportion of the total community nurse-work force consists of hospital assistant nurses.

Table 1.5
Number of personnel employed by the White-Yellow Cross in
1985, 1986, 1989 and 1990, including part-time employees

	1985	1986	1989	1990
head nurses	175	186	225	257
nurses:	2900	3428	4689	4704
of which:				
- graduate	40%	39%	38%	37%
- brevetted	51%	52%	55%	57%
- hospital ass.	10%	9%	7%	7%
administrative personnel**	271	259	351	341
management**	24	36	65	62

Sources: year reports Wit-Gele Kruis, 1985, 1986, 1989; questionnaire

** 1985, 1986, 1990: excluding National level
1989: including National level in the organization

As was noted earlier, the White-Yellow Cross is not the only provider of curative care in Belgium. According to the Ministry of Finance there were 1428 independent nurses in 1987 (Schoofs, 1990) and 4099 contracted by the White-Yellow Cross. In addition to these, there are also nurses working for other organizations, for example Solidarity for the Family.

Manpower Solidarity for the Family The organization started in 1980 with 5 nurses but developed rapidly afterwards, especially in the second half of the 1980s. In 1990 a total number of 1205 nurses was working for Solidarity

(Table 1.6). For every 20 nurses there is one head nurse.

Table 1.6
Nursing personnel employed by Solidarity for the Family in 1990

social nurses (head nurses)	7
graduate nurses	27
brevetted nurses	75
hospital assistant nurses	11
total	120

Source: questionnaire

In 1990 the organization employed 991 home helps (mainly part-timers). Within this type of personnel a distinction is made between home helps with only housekeeping tasks, who are mainly recruited from unemployed women on the one hand and home helps who take care of hygienic and other personal care and psychological support as well, who have had some kind of training in this field on the other hand (Table 1.7).

Table 1.7
Home help personnel employed by Solidarity for the Family in 1990

home help (housekeeping only)	430
home help with hygienic care and psychological support	561

Source: Solidariteit voor het Gezin, 1991

Manpower Child and Family Preventive care is mainly provided by social nurses. Table 1.8 shows the work force of social nurses was quite stable during the 1980s, though the last 4 years show some decline. The relative growth of the number of part-time personnel during the eighties is not visible in the table however. This would have made the decline in manpower more clear.

In addition to social nurses 398 other personnel were employed by Child and Family in 1989.

Table 1.8
Number of social nurses in Flanders during the 1980s,
index figure (1980=100) between brackets

	no of nurses	index figure (1980=100)
1980	785	(100)
1981	724	(92)
1982	785	(100)
1983	750	(96)
1984	789	(101)
1985	789	(101)
1986	708	(90)
1987	768	(97)
1988	703	(90)
1989	676	(86)

Source: Kind en Gezin, 1990

Generally speaking, each nurse takes care of the whole range of activities within the mother and child care sector, including antenatal care, neonatal care and child health care.

Patient populations

White-Yellow Cross The total number of patients cared for during a month in 1990 was 85.000. Of these 85% were chronic patients and 15% were short-term patients (Source: questionnaire).

The size of the population served by a recognized co-operation initiative (see page 18) in home care in Flanders is 25,000 inhabitants. In Flanders there are about 47 of these initiatives. The requisites for recognition do not state a maximum or minimum number of personnel participating in a co-operation initiative.

Table 1.9 clearly shows the high proportion of elderly people cared for by the White-Yellow Cross. Almost 70% are above 70 years of age. It was estimated that 20 to 25% of all patients belonged to the dependent and very dependent group (see page 18).

Table 1.9

**Characteristics of patients cared for by community nurses
of the White-Yellow Cross**

residence	age groups cared for by White-Yellow Cross as % of total number of patients		patient categories according to ADL dependency score (7 point scale)	
- home	0-10	.40	ADL score	
	10-19	.74	1 (min)	50%
	20-29	1.03	2	17%
	30-39	2.37	3	10%
	40-49	3.23	4	10%
	50-59	7.56	5	6%
	60-69	16.5	7 (max)	7%
	70-79	31.81		
	80-	36.37		

		100%		

Source: Geys and Van Loon, 1990

About 75% of all patients receive only nursing care, about 25% receive nursing and home help care, and 1 to 3% receive nursing and social work (Lemaire et al., 1990).

Generally speaking, nurses in the White-Yellow Cross have not specialized in care for specific types of patients nor in specific types of care. By law, brevetted and graduate nurses are considered equals in terms of levels of expertise. Hospital assistant nurses may do the same things as the other nurses, except that they must always be supervised by a brevetted or graduate nurse.

Solidarity for the Family The data collected by Solidarity about the patient population of nursing services resemble the data from the White-Yellow Cross very much and will therefore not be shown.

Figures are available on age for clients of home help services (Table 1.10). Not surprisingly the percentages appear to look very much like those of the users of community nursing care.

Table 1.10
Age of home help clients of Solidarity

age

0-60	10%
60-70	18%
70-80	37%
80-	48%

Source: Solidarity for the Family, 1991

Child and Family The patient population served by Child and Family consists of (expectant) mothers and young children. The children are usually between 0 to 3 years of age. This age group accounts for 90% of the total number of children registered with Child and Family (164,032 in 1988) (Kind en Gezin, 1990). The care can be continued until the sixth year (Commissariaat-Generaal, 1990) if parents think this is necessary for whatever reason or if the social nurse thinks this is necessary. At some consultation bureaus, vaccinations are usually repeated after the third year (Source: questionnaire).

Types of care

White-Yellow Cross Table 1.11 gives an overview of the tasks performed by nurses in the White-Yellow Cross.

Table 1.11
Tasks of nurses in the White-Yellow Cross

- hygienic and other personal care, like bathing, help with lavatory, Activities of Daily Living
- routine technical nursing procedures like injections, catheterization, dressings, stoma, bladder washouts
- more complicated technical nursing procedures like epidural anaesthesia, handling respirator
- psychosocial activities
- encourage help from family members (is done in only 0.1 percent of all home visits (Geys and Van Loon, 1989)
- assessment of individual patient need (this has become more important since the new funding system was introduced on April 1 1991. Before that assessment was exclusively done by GPs)

The Royal Decree of June 18, 1990 is more specific about the technical nursing procedures that may be carried out by nurses. In this decree a distinction is made between activities without doctor's orders and activities for which doctor's orders are needed.

Nurses of each type spend 93% of their total time on home visits (according to questionnaire). There are no consultation hours. The average length of a home visit is 19 minutes (maximum 21, minimum 16) (Geys and Van Loon, 1989). About 5% is spent on paperwork and 2% on visits to homes for the elderly (see Table 1.12).

Table 1.12
Percentage of time spent on selected activities by nurses (all types) in the White-Yellow Cross

home visits	93%
paperwork	5%
visits elderly persons homes	2%

Source: questionnaire

Table 1.13
Number of activities during 1000 home visits (reimbursable activities in italics)

ADL assistance	*433*
subcutaneous injection	*305*
single wound dressing	*128*
intramuscular injection	*127*
eyedrops without dressing	41
multiple wound dressing	*34*
preparing medicine	33
complex wound dressing	*31*
putting patient to bed	24
applying ointment	19
putting on/taking off elastic stockings	16
dressing	14
bladder washout	*6*
blood pressure	5
blood/ urine test with stix	5
other	94
total number of activities during 1,000 home visits	1,315

Source: Geys and Van Loon, 1989

Table 1.13 lists the most important activities during home visits. According to Voskuilen (1991) the reimbursement system (before April 1991) in Belgium strongly favours technical nursing activities (at least compared to the Netherlands), at the expense of preventive and supporting activities.

Solidarity for the Family The tasks of nurses consist of the following activities (Solidarity for the Family 1991):
- nursing and hygienic care
- health education
- psycho-social support
- maintaining contacts with general practitioner, patient and family
Head nurses (social nurses):
- educating and supporting nursing personnel
- administration
- nursing activities if necessary because of personnel shortages
From estimates in the questionnaire it became clear that there is no differentiation in tasks between brevetted nurses and graduate nurses. Both spend about 15% of their time on paperwork and the rest on home visits. The head nurses spend about 40% of their time on paperwork and 10% of their time on home visits.

Child and Family Antenatal care is delivered
1   in 'consultation bureaus', led by a gynecologist who is assisted by social nurses. The social nurses are employed by Child and Family. In these 'consultation bureaus' information and educative sessions are held for future parents.
2   during home visits by social nurses.

Neonatal care is delivered
1   during visits to women in maternity clinics. More than 95% of the women in these clinics is visited (Kind en Gezin, 1990).
2   during neonatal home visits. Within the first six weeks after delivery an average of 3 visits is delivered for each newborn child.
3   during group sessions for new mothers in child health clinics.

Child health care is delivered
1   in 'consultation bureaus for the young child' (child health clinics). Of all children between 1 and 2 years of age 76% were registered with a consultation bureau. Registered children under 4 years visit the consultation bureau four times a year on average (Kind en Gezin, 1990). During the sessions the children are vaccinated, various screenings are carried out and information and advice is given to the mothers. The sessions are led by pediatricians or 'omnipractici' (GPs) (58% of the

sessions by pediatricians and 42% by omnipractici).
2   home visits.
3   group sessions for young parents.

Table 1.14 shows the time spent on selected activities.

Table 1.14
Percentages of total time spent on selected activities by social nurses

home visits	52.1%
of which: antenatal home visits	0.7%
preventive home visits	51.3%
child health clinic	24.2%
consultation hours	26.2%
paperwork	8.0%

Source: questionnaire

Stages in nursing

White-Yellow Cross In most cases first contacts with patients of the White-Yellow Cross are initiated by the patient him/herself or his/her family (table 1.15). Most self-initiators, however, have a prescription from their GP, which is necessary for reimbursement of all activities except ADL assistance.

Table 1.15
Percentage of patients with whom the first contact is initiated by:

patient him/herself or family	80%
general practitioner	5%
hospital/ nursing home for elderly	15%

Source: questionnaire

After referral by a GP, a graduate nurse, or a brevetted nurse decides how the care is going to be financed (since April 1, 1991). She decides whether it concerns a dependent, a very dependent or an independent patient using standardized forms on which the nurse can indicate the Katz-level of dependency (see page 18). On the same form the level of psychological problems and 'environmental problems' can be indicated.

The regulations on co-operation initiatives previously mentioned (see Wauters, 1990 and see page 29) mention the term 'care-plan' which should at least contain the tasks of nurses, GPs and social workers. However, the regulations are very vague in respect of who should make this plan and in what cases. Should it for instance be done for all patients or only for those in need of more than one professional carer?

From expert-information it became clear that, in general, nurses are the ones who decide what care is going to be delivered. It was already indicated that nurses work in a specific geographical area and therefore the decision as to who is going to deliver the care is determined by the area in which the patient lives.

Solidarity for the Family The (estimated) percentages indicating who initiated the first contact with Solidarity's community nursing service are somewhat different from those of the White-Yellow Cross (Table 1.16).

The most remarkable difference is in the large proportion of Solidarity patients whose contact was initiated by the general practitioner (20% vs. 5%).

Table 1.16
Percentage of patients with whom the first contact is initiated by:

patient's family	40%
patient him/herself	25%
general practitioner	20%
home help service	5%
hospital or home for the elderly	10%

Source: questionnaire

For all activities (except ADL assistance) a prescription of the general practitioner is needed, and therefore it is he who decides what care is going to be given. The head nurse decides what type of nurse is going to deliver the care.

Evaluation of the care takes place on a regular basis in cases where a patient is cared for by various types of personnel.

Child and Family Table 1.17 shows who initiated the first contact with social nurses. Almost 100% of all contacts are initiated through the maternity clinics. Almost all deliveries take place in maternity clinics.

Table 1.17
Percentage of patients with whom the first contact with
social nurses is initiated by:

client him/herself   2%
maternity clinic   98%

Source: questionnaire

The frequency of visits to the child health centre and of home visits is determined by the social nurse and the physician of the consultation bureau or
maternity clinic.

Relations with general practitioners, home help services and hospitals

White-Yellow Cross   According to Voskuilen (1991) there is co-operation
between GPs and professionals whom they need regularly: social workers,
nurses, psychologists, dietitians, physiotherapists. How often this co-operation
takes place is not known.
   Earlier we mentioned a legal distinction between two types of activities by
law (Koninklijk Besluit, 18 juni 1990, see page 25). Nurses do not need a
GP's order for the first type of activity. They do for the other. Consequently
nurses are dependent on the GP in order to be allowed to carry out certain
procedures. It should be noted here that these regulations have very little to
do with the reimbursement system: reimbursement requires doctor's orders
always except for ADL assistance.
   The number of GPs a nurse has to work with may vary between 2 and 20.
(Source: questionnaire)
   There are some co-operative initiatives that include home help services.
Lemaire et al. (1990) mention 17 organizations with combined services in the
Walloon provinces. The authors also give guidelines for co-operation, suggest
parameters for evaluation and offer forms to facilitate co-operation between
home help services, community nursing and social work. The key to co-
operation appears to be knowing about and respecting each others tasks and
the identification of patients with whom co-ordination is needed. The authors
suggest using the patient profile form previously mentioned and consider the
'highly dependent' category as liable for co-operative arrangements. Co-
ordination itself can be done by either one of the disciplines, as long as it is
the most important one. The co-ordinator can therefore vary from patient to
patient. In Flanders there are 47 such initiatives.
   Nurses usually have to deal with 1 or 2 home help services. One of the problems in co-operation with home help services is the division of tasks,
especially in respect of hygienic activities. (Source: questionnaire)

Table 1.15 showed that about 15% of the patients cared for by the White-Yellow Cross had been referred by hospitals. There seems to be no need for improvement of relations with hospital staff (Source: questionnaire). Liaison nurses do not exist, though some hospital nurses may also work as independent nurses in the community.

Solidarity for the Family   Two co-operative initiatives recognized by the Flemish government are active in Solidarity (Solidarity for the Family 1991). In these initiatives co-operation takes place between:
- the community nursing service of Solidarity
- the home help service of Solidarity
- the centre for social work of the liberal health insurance funds
- the local associations of general practitioners.
In addition to the activities mentioned above, the co-operation initiative:
- maintains contacts with hospitals and nursing homes
- encourages and supports voluntary work
- promotes health education
- provides continuing education.
Each co-operative initiative has a co-ordinator who is contacted if any of the participants mentioned above encounters a 'difficult case'. The co-ordinator contacts all relevant professionals who are consequently invited to the team. During a team meeting (usually taking not longer than 20 minutes) a care plan is made that is attuned to the needs of the patient. During 1990, the patient himself attended these meetings in 50% of the cases.

Child and Family   The system of consultation bureaus implies a close co-operation between GPs/pediatricians and social nurses. The GP leading a consultation bureau may, however, not be the same as the client's own GP and consequently the nurse may have to deal with many GPs outside the consultation bureaus.

Relations with home help services are not very close, but social nurses may refer their clients to these services if needed.

Relations with maternity hospitals are quite well developed considering the fact that almost 100% of all contacts is initiated from there.

In 99% of the maternity clinics in Flanders patients are visited by social nurses. Maternity clinics in Brussels, however, reject these visits because of the relatively large number of physicians there. These physicians think visits by social nurses are not necessary.

Problems

Underperformance   As it is in many other countries, psychosocial activities with elderly and in child health care are considered underperformed. This problem is enhanced by the fact that the nomenclature for home care does not include preventive and supportive activities (Geys and Van Loon, 1989).

The terminally ill seem to be in need of more complicated nursing as well as psychosocial activities.

Personnel shortages There is a shortage of community nurses, though neither the White-Yellow Cross nor Solidarity for the Family has a waiting list. Possible reasons that were mentioned were that it is hard work for little money and that the government is not undertaking to remedy the shortage. Furthermore an increasing number of nurses are starting to work part-time (in Kind en Gezin this was an important reason for the loss of 120 full-time equivalents in 1989).

Specialist versus generalist In Belgium there are separate organizations and different types of nurses for elderly care and child health care. No problems were reported concerning this division of tasks.

Levels of expertise and home helps No problems were reported in respect of the division of tasks between nurses at the first level of expertise and at the second level of expertise. They are authorized to do the same things. There is some confusion about whose task hygienic care is: the home help or the nurse.

Community nursing and general practitioner Home nurses are very dependent on prescriptions by physicians. No problems were reported on this issue.

Hospital and community nursing No problems were reported on the relations between hospital and community nursing organizations. In some cases there seems to be a need for liaison personnel.

Funding According to the Walloon newspaper La Libre Belgique (26 March 1991) the "nomenclature" needs to be adapted to technical innovations in home care and palliative and preventive care should be integrated within it. Furthermore, the newspaper states that the reimbursement per day of care for highly dependent patients is too low.

According to Van Loon (in Het Volk, 26 March 1991) the government has reserved too small a budget for home care.

References

Commissariat-General for International Co-operation - Flemish Community (1990), *Flanders fact-sheet "child and family"*, Brussels.

De Standaard (1991), 'Wit-Gele Kruis acht forfait thuisverplegers aanvaardbaar' [White-Yellow Cross deems lump sums home care acceptable], *De Standaard*, 26 March.

Geys, L., H. Van Loon (1989), *Wat voeren verpleegkundigen uit in de thuisverpleging? Frequentie van verpleegkundige handelingen in het Wit-Gele Kruis; Koncepten en cijfers ter financiering van de thuisverpleging* [What is done by nurses in home nursing? Frequency of nursing activities in the White-Yellow Cross; Concepts and figures for funding home nursing], Nationale Federatie Wit-Gele Kruis, Brussel.

Katz, S., Ford, A.B., Moskowitz, R.W., Jackson, B.A., Jaffe, M.W. (1963), 'Studies of illness in the aged; the index of ADL: a standardized measure of biological and psychosocial function', *Journal of the American Medical Association*, p. 914-919.

Kind en Gezin (1990), *Jaarverslag* [yearreport] 1989, Brussels.

Koninklijk Besluit (1990), [Royal Decree] 18 JUNI.

Koster, M.K., J. Dekker, P.P. Groenewegen (1991), *De positie en opleiding van enkele paramedische beroepen in het Verenigd Koninkrijk, Nederland, de Bondsrepubliek Duitsland en Belgie,* NIVEL, Utrecht.

Lemaire, G., A. Schiffino, H. Van Loon (1990), *Co-ordination des soins et services à domicile: comment s'y prendre,* Fédération Nationale des Associations Croix Jaune et Blanche, Bruxelles.

Loon, H. Van, Geys, L. (1990), *Patiëntenprofielen in de thuisgezondheidszorg* [Patient profiles in home health care], Nationale Federatie van de Wit-Gele Kruisverenigingen.

OECD (1988), *Ageing populations; the social policy implications,* Organisation for economic co-operation and development, Paris.

Rijksinstituut voor Ziekte- en Invaliditeitsverzekering (1990), *Nationale overeenkomst tussen de gegradueerde verpleegsters of de met dezen gelijkgestelden, de vroedvrouwen, de verpleegsters met brevet, de verpleegassistenten/ziekenhuisassistenten of de met dezen gelijkgestelden en de verzekerings instellingen* [National agreement between graduated nurses and other nursing personnel with insurance companies], Brussel: 4 December.

Schepers, R., H. Nys (1985), *De beroepen in de gezondheidszorg* [professions in health care], In: H. Nys, M. Foets and J. Mertens (eds.), Organisatie van de gezondheidszorg in Vlaanderen [Organisation of health care in Flanders, in Dutch] (p. 53-76), Van Loghum Slaterus, Antwerpen.

Schoofs, M-J. (1990), 'De vier basisdisciplines in de thuiszorg' [The four basic disciplines in home care], *Kontakt*, 45, September.

Solidarity for the family (1991), *Jaarverslag 1990,* [Yearrepport] Solidariteit voor het gezin, Gent.

Statistical Yearbook of Norway 1990 (1990), Statistisk sentralbyrå, Oslo-Kongsvinger.

Vandenberghe L. (1984), *Van Nationaal Werk voor Kinderwelzijn naar 'Kind en Gezin'; De groei en ontwikkeling van de kinderzorg in Vlaanderen gedurende de 20e eeuw,* [From National Organisation for Child Welfare to 'Child and Family'; the growth and development of child care in Flanders in the 20th century], Welzijnsgids - Organisatie II.B. 1.2, July.

Voskuilen, A.H.M. (1991), *Thuisverpleging in Nederland en België;* afstudeerscriptie gezondheidswetenschappen [Home Care in the Netherlands and Belgium, summary in English), Netherlands Institute of Primary Health Care, Utrecht.

Wauters, M. (1991), 'Thuisverpleging in Vlaanderen: op een nieuwe leest geschoeid? Overzicht van de nieuwe relementering van 21 december 1990' [Home nursing in Flanders (..): overview of new regulations of December 21], Kontakt, 47, March.

Wit Gele Kruis van België (1990), *Jaarverslag 1989* [Yearreport 1989], Brussels.

Notes

1. Co-author of this paragraph is drs. Paul van der Heijden.

2. Sources: Statistical Yearbook of Norway (1990); OECD (1988).

3. Main sources:
    -   D.L. Crombie et al (1990), *The interface study*, The Royal College of General Practitioners, London.
    -   M. Schneider et al (1989), *Gesundheitssysteme in internationalen Vergleich: laufende Berichterstattung für den Bundesminister für Arbeit und Sozialordnung,* BASYS, Augsburg.
    -   A.B.M. Gloerich et al (1989), *Regional variations in hospital admission rates in the Netherlands, Belgium and the North of France: basic information and references,* NIVEL, Utrecht.
    -   A. Voskuilen (1991), *Thuisverpleging in Nederland en België,* NIVEL, Utrecht.

4. These figures were given by telephone, by the Belgium Ministry of Health.

2 Community nursing in Canada

The setting

Population

*   total population (1987)   25,7 million
*   % over 65 (1986)   10,7
*   % over 65 (2000, projected)   12,8
*   % over 65 (2010, projected)   14,6
*   % over 65 (2020, projected)   18,6
*   % under 15 (1986)   21,3
*   life expectancy at birth (years) (1987)   71,9 (men)
                                                    79,0 (women)
*   live births (1987) per 1000 inhabitants   14,4
*   population density per sq. kilometre (1987)   3
*   population groups: Canada is a bilingual country, with French being the official language in Quebec and English in the rest of the country. Besides the 'ancient' French and English, there are many minorities from other European countries, and of course one of native Indians (Hatcher et al., 1984) (Sources: Statistical Yearbook of Norway, 1990; OECD, 1988).

Health care system

Introduction Canada's health care program is organized on a federal basis with the provinces responsible for establishing their own health and education policies and services within nationally determined parameters. There are 10 provinces and 2 northern territories (which are directly administered by the Federal Government). Due to their relative independence, there are considerable differences between the provinces. In the province of Alberta,

35

for example, it was allowed to ask a patient for some out of pocket payment, while in other provinces it was not, in spite of the fact that the federal Canada Health Act precludes it (Palley, 1987).

Health insurance According to the Canadian Health Act of 1984 all Canadians are insured for all kinds of health care against no direct costs (Palley, 1987). There is a very small private insurance sector for supplementary insurance.

Funding The provinces are paid a sum of money by the Federal government to organize their health care services. This sum is dependent on the number of inhabitants in that province, but also on the wealth of the province (Palley, 1987). In general 50% of the costs of health care are born by the federal government, but this percentage is diminishing (Source: questionnaire).
   The development of the total expenditure on health in Canada is shown in table 2.1.

Table 2.1
Total and public expenditure on health in Canada (percent of GDP)

year	total expend. % GNP	public expend. % GDP	expend. in Can $ per head
1980	7.36	5.52	941
1981	7.52	5.70	1092
1982	8.37	6.37	1262
1983	8.62	6.57	1391
1984	8.46	6.35	1485
1985	8.50	6.35	1592
1986	8.77	6.53	1745
1987	8.69	6.42	1866

Source: Program ECO-SANTE, BASYS/CREDES

General practitioners In 1988 there were 26,079 general practitioners or family physicians in Canada. This number accounted for one general practitioner per 1,001 inhabitants (Minister of Supply and Services Canada, 1990). General practitioners have access to hospital facilities, admit their patients to hospital facilities and care for them there (Hatcher et al., 1984).
Physicians are paid on a fixed fee-for-service basis with negotiated schedules.

Institutional care The mean length of stay in somatic hospitals in days (1980) (OECD 1987) was 10.7. Referral by a physician, usually a specialist, is needed for hospital admission.

Table 2.2
Inpatient medical care beds and personnel per bed

year	beds total	beds per 1000	personnel per bed
1980	158868	6.6	2.10
1981	161048	6.6	2.13
1982	166020	6.7	2.12
1983	167721	6.7	2.10
1984	169361	6.7	2.14
1985	170523	6.7	2.16
1986	170670	6.7	2.23
1987	171928	6.7	2.25

Source : Program ECO-SANTE, BASYS/CREDES

Community nursing

Canadian provinces are responsible for establishing their own health policies. Community nursing is no exception to this and consequently there are in fact twelve ways of organising community nursing in Canada. The federal government does provide a fixed per capita amount of funding to assist the provinces to provide all health services and the provinces are free to determine the amount spent on community care and all other types of care. Each province has its own system of organising community care and public health. In most provinces community care and public health services (preventive care) operate separately. This is for example the case in Ontario. In Quebec, however, the government established local community health centres for preventive as wel as direct patient care, staffed by a range of professionals including nurses, physicians, social workers, therapists, etc. (Pringle, 1989). In the province of New Brunswick community nursing care is delivered from 'Extramural Hospitals' that provide a comprehensive continuum of services (Steward, 1984) in addition to other community care providers.

The following description of community nursing will be partly based on services provided by the Victorian Order of Nurses, which is the largest non-governmental organization for home care services with branches in 9 provinces (Pringle, 1989).

Because there are considerable differences between the provinces the authors had to make a choice, the following will largely be based on the situation in Ontario.

Another part of this description will be based on information from the St. John's District Health Unit in Newfoundland, a governmental organization which is mainly concerned with public health nursing.

History

Victorian Order of Nurses The Victorian Order of Nurses was created in 1897 to provide care in the home to the sick and dying and to women during childbearing in cities as well as in rural areas. The organization provided preventive as well as direct care services. Until 1975 there were no provincial branches. Each local branch managed financing itself. Governments began to develop insured home care services and contracted with VON to provide nursing services. The provinces control health in Canada so it was necessary to develop a mechanism to negotiate with governments for fees rather than having each local branch conduct its own negotiations. Therefore a provincial board was established and Provincial Executive Directors hired (Source: questionnaire).

St. John's & District Health Unit Prior to 1980 all community public health matters in the province of Newfoundland/Labrador were taken care of by a central headquarters. To increase the regional ability to meet health needs in local communities the province was divided into five Regional Health Units (Source: questionnaire)

Organization and funding

Organization Victorian Order of Nurses The Victorian Order of Nurses is a non-profit, voluntary, charitable organization with units at the local, the provincial and the federal or national level:

federal/national level:	Board of Directors that sets policy for the whole organization and consists of an executive director and directors of Clinical Practice, Communications, Finance and Human Relations.
	Consultation to local branches is provided at this level.
provincial level (9 provinces):	Board of Directors and Executive Director which deals with provincial government and co-ordinates services across branches.

38

local level (73):   73 Units (branches) in 9 provinces. More densely
                            populated provinces have more branches. Each
                            branch has its own geographic boundary. Each
                            branch has a voluntary board that makes policy
                            decisions and to whom the Executive Director
                            (chief nurse) has to report. Each branch has its own
                            charter of incorporation and receives funds to pay
                            for services. Each branch must be financially
                            independent.

Figure 2.1 Organization of the Victorian Order of Nurses in Canada

Four types of nurses are working in VON services (see page 40/41):
- clinical nurse specialists
- public health nurses
- registered nurses
- registered nursing assistants

Besides nursing personnel there are in some provinces home health aides
employed by VON. This is, however, not the case in Ontario.

Specialist knowledge is available at the local level through nurse specialists.
At the national level there are teams of nurses who have developed specialized skills and who, with the director of clinical practice contribute to
program development. These nurses are recruited from the local branches.

The VON premises can be reached 24 hours a day and care is delivered
during nights and weekends if necessary.

Nurses almost always are assigned to geographic districts in which they
provide all the necessary nursing care. However, according to Pringle (1989),
there is an increasing pressure to move to a system of specialized teams, for
instance for palliative care and respiratory care and dementia management
teams. In densely populated areas such teams are already active. The generalist nurses, however, are still responsible for cases without specialist needs.

Organization St. John's & District Health Unit The St. John's and District
Health Unit is a government funded and administered organization directed
toward the prevention of disease, the promotion of healthy lifestyles and the
protection from environmental hazards in St. John's and surrounding areas.

Head of the organization is the Medical Health Officer who carries the
responsibility for six administrative divisions:
1   Public Health Nursing Services
2   Public Health Inspection Services
3   Administrative Support Services

4   Epidemiology and Disease Control
5   Health Promotion
6   Family Health
The organization is staffed by public health nurses, public health inspectors, a health educator, a nutritionist, a social worker and administrative personnel. The nurses work as a team conferencing on clients but operating individually each being individually assigned to a patient.

The organization is available by telephone during office hours but services are available after office hours and on weekends if necessary.

Funding   Community nursing services of VON are funded for 95% by provincial and federal taxes (table 2.3). Provincial as well as federal taxes are paid through the provincial government.

Table 2.3
Sources of income of local branches of the VON services

federal taxes and provincial taxes	95%
private insurance companies	1-2%
donations	2-3%

Source: questionnaire

Out of pocket payment is not required for nursing services.

In some communities in Ontario the contract with the provincial government is split among VON and other agencies of which some are for-profit so that there is some competition between organizations. In the other provinces in which VON branches are active there is some competition with government employed nurses of 'official home care agencies'.

For-profit agencies do not play a significant role in the provision of nursing care in the community but this is not true for the homemaking sector (Pringle, 1989). Nurses are paid a salary by the local branches they work for.

The St. John's and District Health Unit is fully funded through government funds. Public health nurses have an annual starting salary of CD 32,181 and public health nurse co-ordinators of CD 34,747. (Source: questionnaire)

Types of community nurses and manpower

Education   There are four types of nurses employed by VON branches:
-    clinical nurse specialist who (after 5 years highschool) have had a 4 year university education to become a Bachelor of Science in nursing and another 2 years to become a Master of Science in nursing
-    public health nurses who (after 5 years highschool) have had a 4 year

40

university education to become a Bachelor of Science in nursing.
- registered nurses who (after 4 or 5 years highschool) have had a 2-3 year course in a community college leading to a diploma.
- registered nursing assistants who (after 4 years highschool) have had a 10 months community college leading to a certificate.

The St. John's organization employs two types of Public Health Nurses:
- public health nurses with a 3 year hospital diploma plus 1 year speciality in Community Health Nursing and
- public health nurses with a 4 year university program.

According to Pringle (1989) the bachelors degree is increasingly replacing the diploma as the common preparation. It is questioned by some governments whether this is a desirable trend and if an academic degree is really necessary to undertake the responsibilities involved in home care nursing.

Another problematic issue appears to be that nurses in the preventive sector (public health nurses) are moving increasingly to program planning for groups and communities and away from individual work with clients. This requires a different kind of preparation than is given now and which is still focused on working with individual clients of all age groups (Pringle, 1989).

A third educational issue concerns the other registered nurses, not primarily concerned with preventive care. 'Here the dilemma is in the form of generalist versus specialist preparation and organization of services' (ibid).

Manpower No statistics were available on the total number of VON community nurses in Canada or Ontario. The number of personnel is determined by the local branches themselves.

The St. John's organization has two urban offices with 14 public health nurses per office, besides supervisory nursing personnel, health inspection officers, secretarial support, a nutritionist and a health educator. In six rural offices there is a total number of 13 nurses assisted by one registered nursing assistant.

For every 2 public health nurses there are approximately 3,000 inhabitants (Source: questionnaire).

Patient populations

Victorian Order of Nurses Table 2.4 shows age and disease characteristics of patients discharged from VON services during one year (March 1989 - April 1990). Patients over 65 account for 64% of the total patient population and for 73% of the total number of visits. The most prevalent diseases are neoplasms and diseases of the circulatory system (mainly heart diseases). Patients are only cared for at home.

Table 2.4
Characteristics of VON patients (N=101,122) in Canada
(figures refer only to patients that are discharged from VON services)

disease classification		age	
Infective	1%	0-14	4%
Neoplasms	15%	15-44	14%
Metabolic	6%	45-64	18%
Blood disease	1%	65-74	23%
Mental	2%	75-84	28%
Nervous syst.	8%	85+	
Circulatory syst.	16%	13%	
Respiratory syst.	5%		
Digestive syst.	8%		
Genito-urinary	3%		
Skin disease	7%		
Musculoskeletal	7%		
Injury/poison	1%		
Newborn	1%		

Source: questionnaire

St. John's & District Health Unit No statistics appeared to be available on the patient populations in the St. John's organization. It may, however, be assumed that most of the workload concerns children. In the Adult Health Program patients are entitled to one visit per day but exceptions are made based on the patient's condition.

Types of care

Victorian Order of Nurses VON Canada provides various services. Not all services, however, are available in all branches. In Ontario, for example, there are no home making services provided by the VON in most branches.
- visiting nurse services (provided by nurses)
- adult day care (provided by volunteers)
- home making services (provided by homemakers)
- meals on Wheels (provided by volunteers)
- volunteer Visiting
- occupational Health
- senior Citizens Counselling
- footcare
- hospice care, respite care (provided by trained workers)

Within the visiting nurse services all types of care are delivered. The maximum number of visits varies from province to province and from community to community. In Ontario there is a maximum of 3-4 visits a day for a limited period of time (limited is not defined), after which 1-2 visits per day is usually the maximum. The maximum of 3-4 visits applies to terminally ill patients and patients with very acute illnesses who would otherwise be hospitalized. Sometimes there are volunteers (called 'friendly visitors)' available for watching services.

Clinical nurse specialists care for any type of patient, dependent on their specialism. Registered nurses usually work as generalists caring for any kind of patient and delivering any kind of nursing care. Health promotion and assessment of groups at risk is the task of public health nurses. Registered nurse assistants care mainly for the stable patients providing mainly hygienic care.

Table 2.5 gives the percentages of time spent on selected activities by all kinds of nurses. The clinical specialists spend quite little time on home visits and more on consultation hours for their colleagues. As is the case in most countries, nurse assistants spend a relatively small amount of time on paper work.

Table 2.5
Percentage of time spent on selected activities (rough estimates)

	home visits	consult. hours	paper work
clinical specialist nurses	25%	50-60%	25%
public health nurses	80%	-	20%
registered nurses	80%	-	20%
reg. nurse assistants	95%	-	5%

Source: questionnaire

St. John's & District Health Unit The organization provides mainly preventive services that are categorised into nine programs (derived from brochure St. John's and District Health Unit)

1   Prenatal Program. Providing pregnant women with support and information.
2   Postnatal Program. Providing supportive care for women after hospital discharge connected with delivery. Includes a home visiting program after hospital referral.
3   Early Childhood Program. Sessions in child health clinics to ensure the health of the preschool child through health teaching, immunization,

and the monitoring of physical and behavioral development.

4   School Health Program. Includes screening programs, health education and promotion activites, individual counselling with students and monitoring of the school health environment.

5   Adolescent Health Counselling Service. Providing counselling and treatment services for adolescents between 12 and 19 and providing a source of information for persons involved in adolescent health care.

6   Communicable Disease Control.

7   Public Health Inspection. Controlling and inspecting factors in the environment which cause illnesses.

8   Community Nutrition. Promoting good nutrition.

9   Adult Health Program. Providing health promotion for adults and home nursing on a limited basis to disabled and convalescent individuals.

10   Health Education. Providing a variety of media for communicating health messages, including open forums, workshops, mass media and brochures.

No figures appeared to be available concerning the amount of time spent on selected activities. All kinds of nursing tasks are performed by public health nurses. The auxiliaries, however are mainly concerned with assisting the public health nurse and monitoring. They are usually not concerned with technical nursing activities like injections.

Stages in nursing

Victorian Order of Nurses Almost all (99%) patients come into contact with VON services through a home care co-ordinator, who is almost always a nurse, who is appointed by the local administration to co-ordinate home care and who is often hospital based. Being hospital based does not mean that she only refers patients from hospitals. Patients may be referred from home as well.

The home care co-ordinator refers to the VON intake worker. The home care co-ordinator may also refer to home help services, using a limited check list. It is also her task to propose the frequency of visits and when they should be evaluated (the frequency of evaluation varies from branch to branch but is usually monthly). A VON nurse can challenge the home care co-ordinator's decision on the basis of her own assessment. The supervisor of the VON branch decides if the nurse of the district in which the patient lives can provide the care.

Pringle (1989) reports a growing need to develop a comprehensive and uniform assessment and planning process based on an agreed upon philosophy and goal for care.

Each nurse is responsible for her own actions.

St. John's & District Health Unit No figures were available on who initiates the contacts with the organization. On the basis of the fact that most of the services delivered are concerned with mother and child care, we can easily assume that many of the patients will be referred from maternity hospitals. The public health nurse determines the need for care and refers the patient to other organizations if necessary. Each new visit, the care delivered and the patient's need are evaluated by the nurse. Standard forms are used for assessment and screening.

Each nurse is responsible for her own activities and the care she delegates to other health care providers.

Relations with general practitioners, home help services and hospitals

Victorian Order of Nurses VON branches maintain relationships with home care programs, homemaker agencies, family physicians, physio- and occupational therapist agencies.

Contacts with General Practitioners usually take place by telephone, to inform him/her of the patient's condition, to discuss a problem, to recommend a course of action, to seek an order for a medication or activity. In addition, nurses write progress reports every month on every patient to physicians. An individual nurse may have to deal with 15 to 20 or more physicians.

There is very little contact between VON nurses and homemaker services. The home care co-ordinator does most of the 'co-operating' and he or she is informed if the homemaker is not liked by the patient or if the patient complains about the work that is done. In small communities an individual nurse may have to deal with only one homemaking service; in large communities there may be up to 6 or 8 services involved. It should be remembered that there is a large for-profit sector in homemaking.

Contacts with hospitals take place through the home care co-ordinator, who is in many cases hospital based.

St. John's & District Health Unit The organization co-operates with physicians, the Departement of Social Services, school staff, hospital referral nurses, liaison nurses, and other home care agencies.

Public health nurses have ongoing consultation with general practitioners and other physicians dependent on the need for consultation. There are no regular meetings. Nurses in rural areas have to deal with 1 or 2 GPs. In urban areas there may be many more GPs.

Nurses may refer patients to the Department of Social Services for social work assessment and closely co-operate with home help services.

Most hospitals have liaison nurses. They do not deliver care to patients themselves but see to it that information is transferred to the community nursing organizations and that continuity of care is secured.

Problems

Underperformance Also in Canada there seems to be a need for more psychosocial activities and home help care with elderly patients, among whom the mentally ill have a need for more hygienic care as well. More complicated technical nursing procedures are needed by the patients discharged from hospitals. The elderly population needs identification of groups at risk as well.

Personnel shortages Though there is a shortage of community nurses, VON services usually do not have a waiting list. The shortage is due to the rapidly growing need for services and the fact that nurses are better paid in hospitals.

Specialist versus generalist The increase of patients that require specific nursing techniques causes the dilemma between a specialist and a generalist method of working. There is an increasing pressure towards working with specialised teams.

Levels of expertise and home helps According to Pringle (1989), many provinces question the desirability of the tendency of more and more nurses having an academic degree. Is this really necessary to undertake the responsibilities involved in home care nursing?
  The division of tasks between home helps and community nurses was not reported to be a serious problem, though there is a need for more uniform assessment procedures. In Ontario most of the co-ordinating with home help services is done by a home care co-ordinator.

Community nursing and general practitioner/physician No problems were reported in this respect.

Hospital and community nursing The communication and co-ordination with hospitals in Ontario is also the task of the home care co-ordinator. In St. John's there are liaison nurses. No problems were reported in this respect.

Funding Two problems relating to financial matters were reported. First, there is a growing competition from for-profit agencies in an area that historically has been exclusively in the non-profit arena. Furthermore the tight and fixed budgets do not allow for expansion when greater needs are identified.

Other problems The education of public health nurses is not sufficiently adapted to the fact that these nurses are increasingly involved in program planning for groups and communities, instead of working with individual clients.

In Ontario the great influence of the home care co-ordinator is considered to erode the nurses' autonomy.

Nurses are increasingly organizing themselves in trade unions (see Coburn, 1988). This requires more expertise in the field of labour relations.

References

Coburn, D (1988),'The development of Canadian nursing: professionalisation and proletarianisation', *International Journal of Health Services,* 18, 3.

Hatcher, G.H., P.R. Hatcher, E.C. Hatcher (1984), *Health Services in Canada,* In: M.W. Raffel, Comparative Health Systems; Descriptive analysis of fourteen National Health Systems, The Pennsylvania State University.

Minister of supply and services Canada (1990), Health personnel in Canada, Ottawa.

OECD (1988), *Ageing Populations; the social policy implications,* Organization for economic co-operation and development, Paris.

Palley, H.A. (1987), 'Canadian federalism and the Canadian health care program: A comparison of Ontario and Quebec', *International Journal of Health Services,* 17, 4.

Pringle, D.M. (1989), *Community Nursing in Canada,* In: A. Kerkstra and R. Verheij (eds.), Community Nursing; proceedings of the International Conference on Community Nursing, 16-17 March 1989, NIVEL, Utrecht.

Statistical Yearbook of Norway 1990 (1990), Statistisk Senrtralbyrå, Oslo-Kongsvinger.

Steward, J. (1984), *Moving from institutional to community-based services,* Paper presented to the annual meeting of the Canadian Hospital Association, June 15.

3 Community nursing in Finland

The setting

Population
* total population (1987)   4,9 million
* % over 65 (1989)   13,1
* % over 65 (2000, projected)   14,4
* % over 65 (2010, projected)   16,8
* % over 65 (2020, projected)   21,7
* % under 15 (1989)   19,4
* life expectancy at birth (years)   70,7 (men)
                                                         78,7 (women)
* live births per 1000 inhabitants (1988)   12,8
* population density per sq. kilometre (1987)   15
* population groups: there is a Swedish speaking minority. No substantial other minorities (Sources: Statistical Yearbook of Norway, 1990; OECD, 1988).

Health care system

Introduction   Officially Finland is a bilingual country, with a recognized Swedish speaking minority, mainly on the southwest coast. Governmental bodies at all levels have considerable influence on everyday life.

As in the other Scandinavian countries, the organization of health care is the responsibility of governmental bodies. Planning takes place using 5-year plans. In the first stage of this planning, directives are made for local planning. The second stage is the preparation of a local health care plan. Consequently, the local plan will be approved by the regional level and implemented in the local community (Groenewegen et al., 1987) (fig. 3.1). The main responsibility of the central government is to take care that areal equity will be achieved (Espoo, 1987).

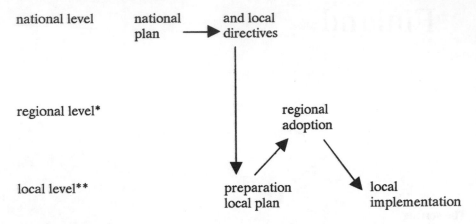

national level   national   and local
               plan ⟶ directives

regional level*   regional
                                  adoption

local level**   preparation   local
                         local plan   implementation

*   11 provinces
** 461 communes, with a total of 217 health centres

Figure 3.1 Customary 5-year planning cycle of primary health and social care in Finland (adapted from Groenewegen et al, 1987)

The state issues three plans: one on primary health care, one for hospitals (excluding health centre hospitals) and one on environmental health care. In 1984 a similar system was adopted for social welfare. (Ministry of Social Affairs and Health, 1987). In 1989 the plans for health care and social welfare were combined and at the moment there is only one plan which includes some common goals and specific chapters for primary health care, hospitals, environmental health care and social welfare.

Primary health care is delivered from health centres, of which there are 217. Large municipalities have a health centre of their own (110) and the smaller municipalities take part in a federation, using one health centre (107). In most cases these health centres employ community nurses, general practitioners, physiotherapists, psychologists, dentists and others. The functions of these health centres are:

- health education
- preventive mental care
- health examinations
- maternal and child health services
- family planning
- school health services
- occupational health (sometimes)
- health services for the elderly

- primary medical and nursing services
- hospitals and sick wards
- dental care
- ambulance service
- laboratory service
- X-ray service
- rehabilitation

50

Usually there is an inpatient department too, which takes care of chronic cases, observation and emergencies. The average number of beds in health centres is about 100.

Health care in municipality based health centres is supplemented by occupational health services which are also part of the general health care system. Its aim is to identify and prevent health risks arising from work or working conditions. Employers may organize the occupational health services themselves or make agreements with the city for providing the services or buy them in a private medical centre (Helsinki City Health Department, 1987). The employer is reimbursed for more than half of the costs of providing such services (ibid.) (55% in 1991). About 12% of all contacts with primary health care take place in occupational health services (Liukko et al., 1991).

Health insurance There is only one, compulsory, health and social insurance system in Finland. It developed from a voluntary unemployment insurance in the 1930s into a fully fledged system covering pensions, sickness, industrial injuries and unemployment for the whole population. Sources of income for the insurance are employer's and employee's premiums, as well as local and national taxes (Crombie et al., 1990).

Primary health care is delivered free of charge. There is, however, co-payment for prescribed drugs. Drugs for chronic diseases are covered for up to 90%, while other medicaments require about 50% out of pocket payment (Ministry of Health and Social Affairs, 1987).

Funding

Table 3.1
Total and public spending on health care (percentage of GDP)

year	total expend. % BNP	public expend. % BNP
1980	6.5	5.1
1987	7.4	5.8

Source: OECD. Health Data File, 1989

General practitioners Most GPs work in health centres and stay there. They rarely make home visits (Crombie et al., 1990). They usually form a group, which, as a group, takes care of a large geographical area. Patients needing a GP make an appointment with any of the GPs in the group, usually with the one that is available soonest.

This, however, has had negative effects on the continuity of care. This and other problems caused the Finnish government to aim at nationwide introduction of the principle of 'personal doctors' in 1990 (Liukko et al., 1990). One of the main characteristics of this principle is that GPs are personally responsible for a more limited geographical area. In this case the municipality is simply divided into areas, each served by one GP. This principle is becoming more and more common in Finland and a research project is currently being carried out to investigate the effects (population responsibility project, see appendix 3, ibid.)

One of the results of the research project is that population responsibility in combination with a different system of remuneration definitely seems to have ameliorated the access and continuity of care. Accessability has increased and waiting lists have become shorter (Liukko et al., 1991). Instead of a waiting list of 2-3 weeks, patients can make an appointment with the GP on the same or next day (ibid.)

GPs are usually paid a fixed monthly salary. In the 'personal doctor' project, however, a new experimental way of remuneration was introduced, to increase the quality of care, as well as to make working in a health centre more attractive. In this experiment the GP's earnings are allowed to vary:
-    60% of his income is based on the number of inhabitants in his area;
-    15% is based on the number of inhabitants in his area who visit a GP 3 or more times a year;
-    10% is based on 'fee for service';
-    5% is based on a GP's special skills, or difficult working conditions.

This new type of remuneration, however, is an experiment and its nationwide introduction is under study.

Institutional care

Table 3.2
Total number of beds and number of beds per 1000 inhabitants

year	beds total	beds per 1000
1980	58599	12.2
1983	59888	12.3
1984	61103	12.5
1985	60958	12.4
1986	60448	12.3
1987	59531	12.1

Source: Yearbook of Nordic Statistics, 1989

Community nursing

Community nursing in Finland is provided by three types of nurses: public health nurses, registered nurses and practical nurses. The first type is concerned with all types of care, both curative and preventive. The second is mainly concerned with curative care and the third is more concerned with the ADL/IADL type of care.

The care is mainly provided from health centres, which take care of a municipality or a group of municipalities.

History

Municipalities have employed nurses since 1879. In 1944 they were obliged to employ communal midwives, public health nurses and doctors. Historically, the main task for nurses was to combat epidemic diseases through vaccinations and health education. The emphasis in their tasks was on preventive activities, but they also delivered acute curative care.

One of the most important landmarks in the history of primary health care in Finland is the 1972 Public Health Care Act. The goal of this Act was to provide for a system that covers the entire population, gives free treatment, aims at equality and endeavours to supply complete but integrated services (Ministry of Social Affairs and Health, 1987). Every community was obliged to provide a health centre, either on its own or with neighbouring community. In Finland a 'Health Centre' does not mean a single building or building complex, but refers to the single organizational entity supplying the services. The act also improved the option of systematic planning at the national, regional and local levels (see page 50) as well as making it easier to diminish regional and socio-economic inequities in the provision of primary health care.

Organization and funding

Organization Community nursing care is delivered from health centres. As we stated earlier, however, the different professions within the health centre are not located usually in the same building. Community nurses may operate from a separate building quite independently.

In many communities health centres and social services, among which the home help services, have the same administration. This is becoming more and more common.

Community nurses usually work from 8.00 to 16.00 h. but they have regular consultation hours in the evenings too. Care can be delivered in the evenings. Urgent cases are cared for at night and weekends and many health centres also have regular community nursing services at night and weekends for patients needing continuous care and support (chronic, terminally ill). Health centers are available by telephone 24 hours a day.

Specialist knowledge can be obtained from specialist nurses or other professionals in the health centres. These specialist nurses are usually also concerned with direct patient care. In fact 'public health nursing' is divided into maternity care, child health care, adult health counselling, school health care, occupational health, domiciliary nursing and ambulatory clinics.' (Helsinki City Health Department, 1988). So there seems to be a lot of specialist knowledge available within primary care, at least in larger cities. It must be noted here that many (about 40%) public health nurses provide more than one of the services mentioned. It is also possible to consult professionals in hospitals if needed.

Large cities are divided into districts, each district with several health stations and a hospital. The city of Helsinki for example is divided into five main districts of about 100,000 inhabitants, each being responsible for primary and ambulatory mental health care in that area (Helsinki City Health Department, 1987). Each main district is divided into primary districts, each with its own health station.

The organization of community nursing is a matter of discussion in Finland. The population responsibility project previously mentioned makes a distinction between three models for public health nursing (Liukko et al., 1990) for which we refer to appendix 3.

Most nurses in Finland work in terms of a specialized model, delivering only one service, e.g. maternal or child care.

Funding Community nursing is part of the local plan which follows the same stages of approval described on page 50.

The health centres are funded by the local as well as national government. National government subsidies are dependent on the wealth of the municipality; on congruity with the national directives; and on the budget requested by the local government. The most prosperous municipalities receive only 35% national subsidies, while in the poorest regions this may be up to 70% (in 1982, Espoo, 1987). The average is a fifty-fifty division of financial burdens between local and central government.

Nursing care is delivered free of charge, although out of pocket payment is required for specific drugs (see page 51). Home help care, however, requires a contribution from the receiver dependent on income. There is no co-payment for low-income families.

Dependent on age and experience a public health nurse has a gross income between 6600 - 9600 FM per month.

Types of community nurses and manpower

General There are three basic types of nurses working in the community in Finland:
- public health nurses
- registered nurses
- practical nurses

Education In 1987 a comprehensive reform of secondary education and training took place in Finland.

All nurses who are trained now have some specialism. Public health nursing is one of the specialisms. Their education varies from 3.5 years to 4.5 years, dependent on previous education. Comprehensive school graduates need 4.5 years, matriculated students 3.5 years. A specialized nurse can continue with studies in universities in order to earn a master's or doctor's degree in health care with public health nursing as a major subject.

Education as a registered nurse (i.e. a nurse generalist) has ceased to exist. The term registered nurse is, however, still used for those who graduated in general nursing before 1987, but also for those who did specialize (after 1987) in a field other than public health.

Becoming a practical nurse takes 1.5 to 2.5 years, also dependent on previous education. About half of all training programs takes place in practical work in the different fields of health care (Liukko et al., 1990).

Manpower Each municipality is free to determine its own staffing ratio. In the city of Helsinki, for example, staffing ratios are calculated by first determining the number of primary health care visits (maternity/child health care, school/student health care, occupational health care) and ambulatory care visits (including home visits) needed for each age group in the population. Then determining the number of visits that *can* be made by each professional, and finally calculating the number of personnel needed (Aho et al., 1987). Therefore these ratios vary locally. National figures do exist, however (Table 3.3).

Table 3.3
Number of inhabitants per nurse (full-time equivalents) in 1986
for nurses working in the community, concerned with direct patient care
(number of full-time equivalents nurses in brackets)

public health nurses	1107 (4487)
registered nurses	4200 (1187)
practical nurses	3903 (1273)

Source: National Statistics, 1989

If we add the number of public health nurses to the number of registered nurses in the community and consider the result as the number of first level nurses in the community, and if we subsequently compare this number with the number of practical nurses in the community (second level), there appear to be almost 4.5 times as many first level nurses as practical nurses.

Patient populations

According to outcomes of the population responsibility project (see above), 27% of the population had used community nursing services during 6 months in 1989. This figure includes home visits as well as consultations in the health centre and includes preventive as well as curative services.

It is impossible to state what patient populations are cared for by what type of nurse in Finland. This varies from community to community. For example in Orivesi, a small town in central Finland, each public health nurse was assigned to a specific area and took care of the whole population in that area, including elderly and maternal health care (the comprehensive model, see appendix 3). On the other hand, in Jyväskylä, a larger town in central Finland there are six public health nurses with specific patient populations in an area: the first takes care of child health care and the elderly, the second mainly antenatal care and some elderly patients, the third and fourth child health care and school health care, the fifth and sixth only do child health care (the semi-comprehensive model).

Table 3.4 shows some characteristics of the patients cared for by all public health nurses. These figures do not refer to any particular specialism, but to all specialisms taken together. Unfortunately, figures for registered nurses and practical nurses are not available. It should be noted that the numbers of elderly, chronically ill, and terminally ill would be much higher if registered nurses and practical nurses had been included. Registered and practical nurses do not care for pregnant women, mothers and the newborn and school children. Furthermore, the figure would be much higher, if we only looked at home nursing: in the city of Helsinki, 80 percent of the patients in home care

are over 75 years of age (Helsinki City Health Department, 1987).

Table 3.4
Characteristics of persons cared for by public health nurses
(all specialisms taken together)

residence	number of patients of public health nurses by age *		category
- home	0-6	22.0%	- pregnant women
	7-14	20.4%	- mothers and new babies
	15-24	9.6%	- mentally handicapped
	25-44	15.7%	- physically handicapped
	45-64	15.5%	- mentally ill
	65-74	9.6%	- terminally ill
	75-	7.3%	- chronically ill
			- post operative
		100%	- adult health care

* figures based on statistics of public health nurses clients in 5 health centres.

Source: population responsibility project

Types of care

It appears from the table above (Table 3.4) that, in Finland, public health nurses care for various types of patients. Many of them, however, have specialized in one type. Usually the emphasis of their workload is on mothers and children. This, of course, is confirmed when we look at the types of care delivered (Table 3.5). It appears from the table that most contacts take place at schools. The high number of contacts may, however, also be due to the fact that visiting a school provides the opportunity to see many children at once. The types of care listed in Table 3.5 include health promotion, assessment of groups at risk, hygienic care, technical nursing procedures, providing information, psychosocial activities, encouragement of help from family members. In some instances also home help care is delivered, but this is mostly done by home help aides, employed by the municipality's social service department and very seldom by registered or practice nurses.

Table 3.5
Types of care delivered by public health nurses in percentages
of the total number of contacts with clients (n=5597*)

maternal health care and birth control	10%
child health care	16%
school health care	38%
adult health care	2%
chronically ill, terminally ill, mental handic.	16%
other	17%

	100%

*   total number of contacts in 9 health centres during one week

Source: population responsibility project

Public health nurses spend very little time on home visits (9% of total working time). Home visits are the task of registered nurses and practice nurses, who, as we stated before, are more concerned with the elderly than public health nurses. Home visits to children and their mothers are rare. Usually the mother is visited at home only one or two times, directly after the delivery. After that mother and child visit the public health nurse once a month during the first year, and once a year until the seventh year. Only 9% of all contacts in child health care concern home visits, and 5% of all contacts in maternal health care.

In general it has to be noted that the division of tasks among public health nurses and between public health nurses and registered nurses as well as practice nurses is a matter of discussion in Finland, and that different solutions are being tried.

Stages in nursing

Results from the population responsibility project (questionnaire to 2099 clients) show that most contacts with public health nurses are established by the patient or by the public health nurse (Table 3.6). The high percentage of contacts initiated by public health nurses is due to the fact that many contacts concern maternal care. After the delivery the public health nurse is informed of the discharge by the hospital and/or she makes an appointment with the expectant mother before the delivery.

Figures on who initiated the *first* contact with public health nurses were not available.

Table 3.6
**Percentage of total number of contacts (N=2111) with public
health nurses initiated by:**

patient's family	4%
patient him/herself	48%
general practitioner	10%
home help, hospital, nursing home, other	6%
public health nurse (sends invitation or previous visit)	32%

	100%

Source: population responsibility project

Assessment is done by public health nurses or registered nurses. They also decide who is going to deliver the care. Usually no checklists are used, though there are guidelines for child health care and maternal health care issued by the National Board of Health. Assessment for home help care and nursing care is not combined, but if the nurse thinks home help care is necessary she can refer the patient.

In general all nurses are responsible for their own actions.

Relations with general practitioners, home help services and hospitals

In most health centres nurses work within a team in which each individual nurse takes care of a specific area. The area can either be defined as a small geographical area or as a certain patient/client group from a larger geographical area. In some areas there are 'areal teams' which have regular meetings and consist of different professional disciplines whose patients live in the same geographical area. In some instances there may be health centre personnel as well as social service personnel taking part in this team.

Generally speaking nurses have regular contact with GP(s) one to four times a month, but of course there is ad hoc contact when needed. Because they work in the same organization, there are good opportunities for contact. Dependent on the size of the area the nurse is working for, she has to co-operate with 1 to 5 GPs.

In Finland home help services and health services have a separate administration. These organizations are also funded differently. Whereas community nursing care is delivered free of charge, there is some out of pocket payment required for home help care. An increasing number of municipalities, however, are integrating the services.

In some municipalities there are regular meetings with home help services (1 to 4 times a month) but it is more usual to have contact only when needed.

There may be 1 to 10 home help aides with whom the nurse co-operates.

In some, mostly sparsely populated, municipalities there is confusion about the division of tasks between nursing and home help. The question is whether simple medication activities always should be the nurse's job, and whether help with instrumental activities of daily living should always be a task for home help aides. In these areas it may be quite uneconomic for different professionals to make home visits to the same patients because of long travelling distances.

Relations with hospitals are sometimes a problem when nurses in health centres feel they do not get enough information from the hospitals. On the basis of information from a Finnish hospital, Saltman (1987) states: 'Health centre visiting nurses still on occasion learned of a patient's impending discharge the same day the patient was due to go home, a decision sometimes made without consideration as to whether adequate home support services would be available'.

Co-operation between hospital and health centre sometimes needs improvement. This is mostly a problem with elderly patients needing both nursing and home help services. Sometimes information about these patients does not reach the health centre in time. However, in the case of maternal care health centres are always informed in time when a mother leaves the hospital.

Problems

Underperformance The following activities were considered underperformed:
-       hygienic and other personal care, psychosocial activities, encouragement of help from family members and home help care for the elderly. Some elderly people have to be taken care of in hospitals because of insufficient resources in ambulatory care;
-       hygienic care and stimulation of help from family members with terminally ill people;
-       psychosocial activities with children and their mothers. Problems in this area are becoming more and more evident. Many nurses feel they do not have the opportunity to shift the focus of the patient contacts from the long list of physical examinations to psychosocial activities.

Personnel shortages Waiting lists do not exist in Finland, though there is a shortage of community nurses in a few areas.

Specialist versus generalist After several years of experience with a specialist method of working (separating for instance preventive care from home nursing), this approach is currently under discussion. The specialist method of working causes an undesired fragmentation of care and decreases the nurses' commitment to the people in the community. On the other hand, the increasing complexity of care calls for specialization.

According to researchers on the population responsibility project, the solution to this dilemma should depend on the local needs of the community, the population density and age distribution.

Levels of experience and home helps The increasing demand for both home help and nursing care leads to higher demands on the quality of the relations between the two disciplines. There is a trend towards more integration between the two services.

No problems were reported on the division of tasks between various levels of community nursing and between community nurses and home helps.

Community nursing and general practitioner No problems were reported in the co-operation between community nurses and general practitioners.

Hospital and community nursing Relations with hospitals are sometimes a problem when community nurses feel they do not receive enough information about patients who are discharged. This is especially a problem with elderly patients needing both home help and community nursing care.

Funding No problems were reported concerning the funding of community nursing care.

References

Aho, S-L., S. Elfving (1987), *Norms set for health care: functions and personnel*, Helsinki.

Crombie, D.L., P. Backer, J. Van Der Zee (1990), *The Interface Study*, EGPRW, Birmingham.

Espoo, A.S. (1987), 'Health expenditure by area in Finland - an indicator of equity', *Health Policy,* 7, pp. 299-315.

Groenewegen, P.P., R. Willemsen (1987), *Naar een sterkere eerste lijn? Part 2: buitenlandse ervaringen,* [Strengthening primary health care? Part 2: experiences abroad], NIVEL, Utrecht.

Helsinki City Health Department (1987), *Health care in the city of Helsinki*, Helsinki.

Helsinki City Health Department (1988), *A change to community nursing*, Handout at Conference on Health Target Challenges to Nursing Practice in Vienna.

Liukko, M., K. Perttilä, S. Aro (1990), *Small area based population responsibility; an action - research approach to reorganize primary care*, Paper issued by National Public Health Institute, Health services research unit, Helsinki.

Liukko, M., K. Perttilä, S. Aro (1991), 'Egenläkarensystem prövas inom Finländsk primärvård', [Personal doctor system tested in Finnish primary care], *Nordisk Medicin*, 106, 4.

Ministry of social affairs and health, National board of health (1987), *Health Care in Finland*, Helsinki.

OECD. *Ageing populations; the social policy implications*, Organization for economic co-operation and development, Paris.

Saltman, R.B. (1987), 'Management control in a publicly planned health system: a case study from Finland', *Health Policy* 8, pp. 283-298.

Statistical yearbook of Norway 1990 (1990), Statistisk Sentralbyrå, Oslo-Kongsvinger.

Statistical Yearbook of Finland (1987), Central statistical Office of Finland, Yearbook of Nordic Statistics 1989 (1990), Nordic Council of Ministers and the Nordic Statistical Secretariat, Stockholm.

4 Community nursing in France

The setting

Population [1]
* total population (1987)   55,6 million
* % over 65 (1989)   13,8
* % over 65 (2000, projected)   15,3
* % over 65 (2010, projected)   16,3
* % over 65 (2020, projected)   19,5
* % under 15 (1989)   20,3
* life expectancy at birth (years) (1987)   72,0 (men)
     80,3 (women)
* live births per 1000 inhabitants (1988)   13,8
* population density per sq. kilometre (1987)   101
* population groups: there are cultural minorities from Mediterranean countries, in part being former French colonies.

Health care system

Introduction The health care system of the republic of France is character-ized by a rather fragmented structure. The central legislative body is the ministry of health. Considerable decision making power is delegated to various health insurance funds. The fragmented structure results in consider-able regional differences in the organization as well as the amount of services offered.

Health insurance [2] There are three main types of insurance in France.
1   Compulsory insurance (Régime Générale) for all employees, pensioners and unemployed persons. The Regime Generale is executed by many local and regional Caisses Assurance Maladie (health insurance funds). These Caisses vary in the amount of premium that has to be paid and the same is true for the benefits. In 1982, 80% of the population was covered by this general scheme.

The insurance is based on the reimbursement principle: the patients pay directly and then claim a refund. According to Collaris and De Klein (1987) the medical costs are reimbursed as follows:
-    75% of the fees of general practitioners and dentists;
-    65% of paramedical treatment;
-    100% or 70% or 40% of the costs of drugs;
-    80% of the costs of the first 30 days of hospital treatment (thereafter 100%);
-    65% of tests and general care.

Copayment is called 'Ticket Moderateur'.
2   Special schemes for agricultural workers, miners, seamen, civil servants and railway employees.
3   Private supplemental insurance (Mutualité): 58% of the population. These insurances re-insure co-payments and cover risks that are not covered by the Régime Générale.

Funding

Table 4.1
Total and public expenditure on health in France (percentage of GDP)

year	total expend. % GDP	public expend. % GDP	expend. in FF per head
1980	7.56	5.95	3938
1981	7.87	6.25	4595
1982	7.97	6.30	5303
1983	8.15	6.35	5964
1984	8.49	6.57	6742
1985	8.45	6.50	7193
1986	8.54	6.49	7762
1987	8.52	6.37	8095

Source: Program ECO-SANTE, BASYS/CREDES

Composition of total health spending:

* total expenditure on institutional health in % of total expenditure on health (1983, from OECD, 1985): 46.2
* total expenditure on ambulatory health services in % of total expenditure on health (1983, from OECD, 1985): 26.0

General practitioners [3] There are 1.25 general practitioners per 1000 inhabitants. Most GPs work in solo practices. They are reimbursed on a fee for service basis by the patients, who are in turn reimbursed by health insurance funds. The patients are not registered with a physician and are free to chose their own doctor. Home visits account for one third of all contacts with patients.

Institutional care [4] A fairly high percentage of all hospitals is in private hands. Some of these private hospitals are for-profit. It is not necessary to have a referral by a GP to obtain specialist care in hospitals or in ambulatory setting.

The mean length of stay in somatic hospitals in days in 1978 was 13.5 (OECD, 1987).

Table 4.2
Inpatient medical care beds and personnel per bed

year	total	beds per 1000	personnel per bed
1980	597800	11.1	1.41
1981	604031	11.1	1.44
1982	601436	11.0	1.48
1983	593867	10.9	1.51
1984	588377	10.7	1.53
1985	579990	10.5	1.56
1986	574612	10.4	1.58
1987	564879	10.2	1.61

Source: Program ECO-SANTE, BASYS/CREDES

Community nursing

Community nursing in France is delivered by a great diversity of organizations. We will concentrate here on the curative services. Preventive (child health care) services are sometimes integrated in organizations for curative community nursing care. Usually, however, they are organised separately.

Generally speaking there are two types of organization for curative community nursing care. One type is organized by municipalities and the other type was brought about by private initiative, mostly non-profit (associations à but non-lucratif). Within these two types there is a large variety in composition of services offered to the public and in the size of organizations. There is a very small number of for-profit organizations. A large part of the community nursing services in France is done by so called 'libérales', independent nurses working on a fee for service basis. Nurses who have a permanent appointment with an organization are not allowed to be involved in direct patient care. They have a co-ordinating role and the direct patient care should be reserved for second level nurses (aides soignantes) with a permanent appointment or for independent (first level) nurses (Source: questionnaire).

Because there is very little general literature on community nursing in France, the following description of community nursing organizations will largely be based on the two organizations that were visited in February 1991: Association Medico Sociale Anne Morgan (AMSAM) in Soissons, northern France and Santé Service Charente (SSC) in Angoulême, southwestern France.

Both are non-profit organizations and founded on private initiative. Though these organizations offer a large variety of services, we will concentrate on the nursing services.

History

Association Médico Sociale Anne Morgan After the first world war the departement of Aisne was a devastated area and in great need of foreign assistance. Foreign assistance came from the United States in the form of money and Miss Morgan. She in fact laid the basis for an organization to 'help populations to help themselves' which consequently developed into the Association Medico Sociale de l'Aisne in 1954. In that year the organization covered home nursing care, social work, and maternal and child health care. In the following years of its existence new services were introduced like a restaurant for elderly and disabled people, together with a meals on wheels service (1958), a home help service (1960), a laundry service (1961), a chain of 'Clubs', for social and cultural activities (1962).

In 1980 a Service de Soins à Domicile aux Personnes Agées (home care service for the elderly, SAD) and a Service d'Hospitalisation à Domicile (hospitalisation at home, HAD) were created. In the years thereafter the most important new developments were the creation of a Télé Alarme Service, and a Service d'Auxiliaires de Vie (assistance with activities of daily living). The existing services were extended (Diebolt and Laurant, 1990).

Santé Service Charente The Santé Service Charente originated in an initiative by the 'departemental' division of the National League against Cancer together with hospital physicians to create a service for patients whose health status did not justify their presence in hospital and for terminal patients whose families wished them to die at home. At first this service was offered only by volunteers but soon salaried personnel was taken on. The Santé Service was created in 1974 as a Service d'Hospitalisation à Domicile (HAD). In 1978 the service was extended with a Service de Soins à Domicile aux Personnes Agées (SAD). In 1982 a new service was introduced: Assistance Ventilatoire à Domicile, providing respiratory equipment at home.

   In 1990 both services (HAD and SAD) have become social services of the departemental health insurance fund (Mutualité de la Charente).
(Source: questionnaire)

Organization and funding

Organisation Association Médico Sociale Anne Morgan Though AMSAM is in fact an independent organization, it has close connections with the local government.
The organization provides a number of services:
.   Service Social Familial Polyvalent (Social services)
.   Protection Maternelle et Infantile (PMI, maternity and child health care)
.   Service de Soins à Domicile (SSD, nursing care at home)
.   Service de Soins à Domicile aux Personnes Agées (SAD, nursing care at home for elderly)
.   Service Hospitalisation à Domicile (HAD, hospitalization at home)
.   Maintien à domicile du 3me âge (home support services for the elderly)
.   Service d'Auxiliaires de Vie (support with activities of daily living)
.   Service Aides Menagères (home help services)
.   Laundry services
.   Clubs
.   Handyman service
.   Telephone alarm service
.   Service gardes domicile nuit et jour (day and night watching service)
In addition to the list above there are some services that are the responsibility of the local government but that are in fact run by AMSAM:
.   Centre de reinsertion (rehabilitation center)
.   Repas à domicile (meals on wheels)
.   Social centers
.   Old age homes
AMSAM can be compared to an octopus with tentacles of varying lengths: the area covered by HAD services is smaller than the area covered by SAD,

the area covered by laundry services is smaller than that covered by the home help services, etc. None of the services of AMSAM cover the whole 'departement' of Aisne. The nursing services of AMSAM cover an area of about 90,000 inhabitants.

Other areas in the 'departement' of Aisne have other organizations. Some parts of the 'departement', however, are not covered at all by certain services. This is a problem especially in rural areas.

Specialist knowledge can be obtained from the school of nursing, school for home helps and organizations like the Centre d'Animation Soins et Services aux Personnes Agées in Soissons, that, among other things, organizes courses for nurses and other personnel.

The organization can be reached 24 hours a day.

Organisation Santé Service Charente There are two large differences between AMSAM and SSC. First, SSC does not offer as many services. Second, SSC covers a whole 'departement'. The services offered by SSC are SAD, HAD and Assistence Ventilatoire à Domicile, which provides respirators at home and is not really a nursing service. Another difference is that both, SAD, HAD and AVD are services provided by the Mutualité de Charente, a regional supplementary insurance company which also provides home help and other services. The 'departement' is serviced by 6 centers, each led by 'infirmieres coordinatrices' (co-ordinating first level nurses) who are responsible for 10 to 20 'aides soignantes' (second level nurses) (Santé Service Charente, 1991). Each 'infirmière' is responsible for about 50 patients, and each 'aide soignante' for about 6 patients per day. In addition to these, an varying number of independent (first level) nurses is employed on a free lance basis. There is no known source of specialist knowledge.

The organization can be reached by telephone between 08.00 and 18.00 hours.

Umbrella organizations There is a variety of regional and national umbrella organizations. Only one of these will be discussed here: Union National des Soins et Services à Domicile (UNASSAD), which can actually be considered an interest group rather than an umbrella organization with decision making power. The most important aim of this organization is, in view of the rapidly growing number of elderly people, to propagate a holistic approach in home care for the elderly population. This is reflected by the list of members of this organization, consisting of home help services, nursing services, telephone alarm services and the like. UNASSAD wants:
- to regroup and co-ordinate departmental structures consisting of local organizations
- to stimulate new initiatives
- to represent personnel to the authorities

-    to create common services that can be used by member-organizations. The most important task, however, is considered to be a change in the funding system, especially for the social and home help services that have an important place in their holistic approach. As it is today, reimbursement of these services is dependent on the 'departement' in which the patient lives, and on the social insurance fund he has. Large regional as well as individual differences exist in this respect and therefore UNASSAD pleads for a 'fonds national pour un veritable soutien à domicile', a national insurance which covers the whole range of home care services.
(Source: UNASSAD, 1991)

As we will see below this plea seems to be have an effect, considering the most recent government publication on dependent elderly people (Assemblée Nationale, 1991).

Funding HAD and SAD are both funded by lump sums. In 1990 this was 305.66 FF. per bed for HAD and 105,75 FF for SAD per patient per day. SSD concerns fee for service. Organizations have to apply individually to health insurance funds to get permission to offer HAD and/or SAD services. The organization then receives authorization to care for a fixed number of 'beds' on which the lump sum is dependent. This number, however, is somewhat theoretical. Patients are not always refused if this number is exceeded. Service Santé Charente, for instance has permission for 125 beds but had 141 patients on the first of January 1990 (Santé Service Charente, 1990).

SSD, which is only registered as such in the statistics of AMSAM, is reimbursed on a fee for service basis according to the 'Nomenclature des actes professionels'. HAD requires a permission/ prescription of the general practitioner and the hospital physician. SSD and SAD require permission/ prescription of the general practitioner or a hospital physician. In addition, for SAD, the patient has to be over 60, though exceptions are made for handicapped people. After written permission, the consulting physician of the patient's insurance company has to give his consent (Source: questionnaires).

There is a large variety of health insurance funds in France and community nursing organizations may have to deal with many of them (5 to 7). In general the obligatory health insurance funds reimburse about 70% (there can be considerable differences between these health insurance funds in this respect) of the costs of community nursing services and the other 30% (ticket moderateur) has to be paid by the patient himself or, if he is additionally insured, by his complementary insurance (Mutualité) (Source: questionnaires).

There is a maximum to the number of visits patients receive. They may receive 4 x 30 minute visits from independent nurses and/or 2 x 1.5 hour visits from aides soignantes. Exceptions are made for terminally ill patients (Source: questionnaire Santé Service Charente).

Recent developments In June 1991, a report was published by the central government in which several measures were proposed to cope with the growing demand for home care for the elderly (Assemblée Nationale, 1991). Earlier we mentioned UNASSAD's campaign for a kind of national insurance for dependent elderly people which would cover the whole range of home care services.

This is roughly what is being proposed in the report of the Assemblée Nationale.

Several proposals have been made:
- to increase the number of places by 45,000;
- to integrate medical and social services, in practice as well as in funding;
- to introduce an 'allocation autonomie et dépendance' in which this new system of reimbursement is regulated;
- to introduce a system of reimbursement in which the reimbursed sum is dependent on the patient's level of dependency. The higher the dependency the higher the sum that is reimbursed;
- to heighten the reimbursement;
- to find resources to fund this new system for entry;
- a shift from long term residential care to home care;
- to encourage informal care by relatives.

These proposals are still under discussion but it is the first government report that makes some quite specific suggestions on funding a better system of services for the dependent elderly.

Types of community nurses and manpower

Education Nurses have had three-year's training at nursing schools. After graduation there are a lot of options for specialization. There is, however, no specialization in community nursing. An eighteen month study is required to become a chief nurse (infirmière co-ordinatrice). The second level nurses are called 'aides soignantes'. They have had one year's training.

Nurses directly employed by an organization receive a gross income of 7.878 FF a month. Aides soignantes 6,745 FF.

Manpower Recent national statistics on total community nursing manpower do not exist. Statistics are kept by individual organizations but they do not cover the number of independent nurses in that area. However, the statistics that do exist suggest a rapid growth in the number of community nurses. Both organizations that were visited showed considerable growth during the last decade in the number of places for HAD and SAD.

The only national statistics that were found were gathered in 1984 (Ministère des Affaires Sociales et de la Solidarité Nationale, 1986) and these only cover the organizations providing SAD, not including all independent nurses. First of all a rapid growth in the number of organizations is noted (from about 50 in 1979 to about 650 in 1984). In 1984, however, there are very large regional differences, differences that, according to Nijkamp et al. (1991) still exist.

Table 4.3 shows the number of nurses in organizations for SAD services in 1984.

Table 4.3
Number of nurses in SAD services in 1984

salaried first level nurses (infirmières)	1400
salaried second level nurses (aides soignantes)	3700
independent nurses (libérales)	2400

Source: Ministère des Affaires Sociales et de la Solidarité Nationale, 1986

Looking at this table, it becomes clear that, within organizations (salaried personnel), there are almost trice as many aides soignantes as there are infirmières.

The organization visited in Angoulême (Santé Service Charente) was a very clear example of many aides soignantes and few infirmières, employing only 13 infirmières and 133 aides soignantes. The task of the first level nurses here is to co-ordinate and maintain relations with other care providers. The aides soignantes take care of the hygienic care, psychosocial care and some home help type care, like shopping. The medical and nursing activities are taken care of by independent nurses who are paid on fee for service basis according to the nomenclature.

In 1988 AMSAM employed 9 first level nurses, 17 second level nurses (aides soignantes) and had contracted 12 independent nurses (libérales).

Patient populations

General The figures on pp. 71 clearly indicate the high percentage of the elderly in the French population. Figures of the "Caisse Nationale Assurance Maladie" presented in the previously mentioned Rapport d'Information (Assemblée Nationale, 1991), indicate that there are at present 38,872 persons above 60 being cared for by home care services. This is about 0,4% of the total population over 60.

Association Médico Sociale Anne Morgan During 1989, 77 patients were cared for under the HAD-scheme. The average length of stay in HAD was 75 days. Table 4.4 shows some characteristics of these patients (Yearreport AMSAM, 1989). A growing number of patients are in the terminal phase of their illness.

Table 4.4
Characteristics of patients receiving HAD from AMSAM 1989

sex	pathology		age	
	cancer	48%		
male: 44%	cardio vasc.	22%	0-60	26%
female: 54%	neurology	17%	60-80	49%
	chirurgy	12%	80-	25%
	polypathology	36%		

Source: AMSAM: Rapport d'activites 1989, Bilan d'activités Hospitalisation à Domicile, 1989

During 1989, 209 patients were cared for under the SAD scheme. The average length of stay in SAD was much longer than in HAD (164 days versus 75 days). Their mean age was also higher: 81 years. This is not surprising since being over 60 is one of the conditions for admission. About 80% of the patients were considered heavily or moderately dependent, the rest was independent or slightly dependent (definitions of these terms are lacking).

It is not known how many patients received SSD and what their characteristics are.

Santé Service Charente In 1990 there were 1003 patients under the HAD scheme (including 306 readmissions). Their average length of stay was 51 days. Table 4.5 shows the characteristics of these patients. Santé Service Charente provides care for people living at home as well as living in 'hèbergements pour personnes agées' (homes for elderly with very limited nursing possibilities).

Table 4.5
Characteristics of patients under HAD in 1990 at
Santé Service Charente (N=1003)

sex	age		medical motif for HAD	
			cancer	31%
male: 43%	0-60	20%	cardio-vasc	21%
female: 57%	60-80	38%	traumato-	
	80-	41%	orthopedics	21%
			neurology	10%

Source: Santé Service Charente, 1991

Comparing patients under the SAD (Table 4.6) with those under the HAD scheme confirms what we already saw with AMSAM. The patients are older and stay longer (135 days versus 51).

Types of care
Figures provided by the Santé Service Charente show that the biggest difference between SAD and HAD is in the number of patients needing technical nursing care (Table 4.7). For example in 68% of the HAD cases injections are given, whereas this is only 34% of the SAD cases. However, during one of the author's visits, it often appeared not to be very easy to see the difference between HAD and SAD care in practice, not even for the nurses themselves.

Table 4.6
Characteristics of patients under SAD in 1990 at Santé Service Charente

sex	age		medical motif for SAD	
male: 35%	0-60	2%	cardiology	12%
female: 65%	60-80	32%	cario-vasc	28%
	80-	67%	neurology	26%
			rheuma	5%
			traumato-	
			orthopedics	13%

Source: Santé Service Charente, 1991

Table 4.7
Nature of interventions, SAD and HAD of the Santé Service Charente in 1990 in percentages total number of patients receiving HAD or SAD

	HAD	SAD
hygienic care	100%	100%
mobilization	81	80
prevention of scab	96	96
getting out of bed	90	95
getting to bed	35	15
technical nursing:		
- injections	68	34
- perfusions	17	6
- blood pressure	16	10
- dressings	30	14
- stoma care	4	0
- catheterization	19	4
- oxygen	3	0
- other	2	1

Source: Santé Service Charente, 1991

As we saw on pp. 75 , the Charente organization works with few nurses (13) and many auxiliaries (133). Table 4.8 clearly shows that their tasks differ greatly. Aides soignantes spend almost twice as much time on visits and their visits are of much longer duration (Santé Service Charente, 1991). It should be remembered, however, that many visits are done by independent nurses, hired by the Service Santé. They take care of 21% of the total number of visits, aides soignantes 71% and the salaried infirmières only 8% (Santé Service Charente, 1991).

Table 4.8
Percentage of time spent on selected activities by salaried personnel in the Santé Service Charente (independent nurses not included)

	travelling	visits	paperwork
infirmières salariées	10%	45%	45%
aides soignantes	16%	80%	4%

Source: Santé Service Charente, 1991

Table 4.9 shows the sources of referral to SAD and HAD in the Service Santé Charente (such statistics were not available for AMSAM). Most of the HAD patients are referred by hospitals, while most of the SAD patients are referred by family, friends, neighbours or by the patient himself. This is not at all surprising since one of the requirements for HAD is to have orders from a hospital physician. For SAD orders from a GP are sufficient. The orders are quite specific concerning what type of care needs to be given, and since hygienic care is by definition given by aides soignantes and technical nursing care by infirmières, the orders also determine who is going to give the care.

Table 4.9
Sources of referral to HAD and SAD in 1990, Santé Service Charente

	HAD	SAD
hospital	52%	11%
general practitioner	10%	14%
family/friends/self	37%	55%
other	1%	2%
HAD	--	18%

Source: Santé Service Charente, 1991

During the period in which the care is delivered a dossier is kept containing background information and a functional assessment form together with records of each visit. The SAD dossiers also contain records of visits by home helps and a list of medical prescriptions. In addition, the HAD dossiers contain records for home helps and nurses, a general list of observations intended to provide a chronological view of treatment and observations by all active professionals. We were informed, however, that not all professionals use the dossier. General practitioners seemed to be a particular problem.
In Service Santé Charente the HAD care is evaluated weekly, the SAD care monthly. AMSAM does not have regulations in this respect.

Relations with general practitioners, home help services and hospitals

Association Médico Sociale Anne Morgan Nursing personnel in AMSAM works with all professionals that are needed with a patient. Nurses may have to work with many general practitioners but only with one organization for home help care: the one that is organized by AMSAM itself. There is no problem concerning the division of tasks between home helps and aides soignantes. There seems to be no need for special nurses to maintain relations with hospitals.

Santé Service Charente   The SSC works with hospitals and independent professionals like general practitioners, independent nurses, physiotherapists and occupational therapists. One of the main tasks of the 13 coordinating nurses working for the SSC is to maintain these relations. Every thirty days admissions and extensions are discussed with general practitioners. There are regular meetings with leading personnel of the home help service, particularly to discuss the number of hours a patient needs to be cared for. The division of tasks between aides soignantes and home helps is not problematical since their tasks are well defined.

A nurse may have to deal with all the home help services in the area they are working in as well as with all general practitioners.

Problems

Underperformance   A need for more of the following activities was reported from both organizations:
-   assessment of groups at risk in the community, for perinatal care users in particular.
-   hygienic care for all patient categories
-   home help care for elderly patients

In addition, a need for more stimulation of informal care; information on for instance medicine or nutrition; and more technical nursing care were reported from AMSAM.

Personnel shortages   Both organizations complain about a shortage of community nurses. Two reasons were mentioned: low payment compared to hospital nurses, and working conditions of nursing in general (difficult to combine it with family life).

The Service Santé has a waiting list of several weeks. The reason for this is the fact that the maximum number of patients that they are authorized to care for is not sufficient. The financial resources based on this number are too small.

AMSAM does not keep a waiting list.

Specialist versus generalist   No problems were reported in respect of the specialist-generalist dilemma.

Levels of experience and home helps There appears to be no discussion about the division of tasks between infirmières and aides soignantes. By definition hygienic care is given by aides soignantes, technical nursing care by independent nurses, and the co-ordination is taken care of by the infirmières coordinatrices.

Furthermore, no problems were reported concerning the division of tasks between aides soignantes and home helps.

Community nursing and general practitioner Home nursing has to be authorized by a general practitioner and (in case of HAD) by a hospital physician. No problems were reported in this respect.

The only problem that appeared during one of the authors' visits, was the fact that general practitioners tend not to state their activities in the patient dossiers.

Hospital and community nursing No problems were reported on the communication between hospital and community nursing organisation.

Funding The community nursing organization has to deal with many health insurance funds. This is sometimes considered a problematical issue. Another problem is that home help and community nursing services are not funded the same way and that there are regional differences.

This, however, is probably going to change in the near future.

Other problems France is not (yet) fully covered by community nursing and home help services. There are regional differences.

References

Assemblé Nationale (1991), *Rapport d'Information N°2135 déposé en appli-
cation de l'article 145 du Règlement par la Commission des affaires
culturelles familiales et sociale sur les personne âgées dépendantes, vivre
ensemble,* Assemblé Nationale, Paris.

Association Médico Sociale Anne Morgan: various information brochures.

Association Médico Sociale Anne Morgan (1989), *Bilan d'activités Hospitalisation à Domicile,* Soissons.

Association Médico Sociale Anne Morgan (1989), *Rapport d'activités,* Soissons.

Crombie, D.L., P. Backer, J. Van Der Zee (1990), *Interface Study,* EGPRW,
Birmingham.

Collaris, J.W.M., C. De Klein (1986), *Sociale ziektekostenverzekeringen in
Europees perspectief: Voorstudies en achtergronden,* Staatsuitgeverij, 's-
Gravenhage.

Diebolt, E., J-P. Laurant (1990), *Anne Morgan; une Américaine en Soissonais
(1917-1952); de l'Aisne dévasté à l'action sociale,* Soissons.

Gloerich, A.B.M., R.T.J. Hamers, J. Van Der Zee, P.P. Groenewegen (1989),
*Regional variation in hospital admission rates in the Netherlands, Belgium,
and the North of France: basic information and references,* NIVEL,
Utrecht.

Ministère des Affaires Sociales et de la Solidarité Nationale (1986), Publication: service des statistiques de études et des systèmes d'information
(SESI), Solidarité Santé; Cahiers Statistiques 8, *Les services de soins
infirmiers à domicile pour personnes agées; caractéristiques-activité-
clientèle 1984,* Paris.

Nijkamp, P., J. Pacolet, H. Spinnewyn, A. Vollering, C. Wilderom, S. Winters
(1991), *Services for the elderly in Europe; A cross-national comparative
study,* Commission for the European Communities, Leuven.

OECD (1988), *Ageing populations; the social policy implications,* Organisation
for economic co-operation and development, Paris.

Santé Service Charante (1991), *Statistiques 1990,* Angoulême.

Santé Service Charante, Various information brochures.

Statistical Yearbook of Norway 1990, 109th issue (1990), Central Bureau of
Statistics, Oslo-Kongsvinger.

Union Nationale des Associations de Soins et Services a Domicile (UNASS-
AD) (1981), Various information brochures.

WHO (1981), *Legislation concerning Nursing/Midwifery Services and Education,* Report on a WHO study, World Health Organization, Regional
Office for Europe, Copenhagen.

Notes

1. Sources: Statistical Yearbook of Norway (1990); OECD (1988).

2. Main source: Gloerich et al (1989).

3. Source: Crombie, Backer and Van der Zee (1990).

4. Source: Crombie, Backer and Van der Zee (1990).

5 Community nursing in Germany (situation before 1990)

The setting [1] [2]

Population [3]

* total population (1987)   61,2 million
* % over 65 (1987)   15,1
* % over 65 (2000, projected)   17,1
* % over 65 (2010, projected)   20,4
* % over 65 (2020, projected)   21,7
* % under 15 (1987)   14,7
* life expectancy at birth (years) (1985/87)   71,8 (men)
                                                         78,4 (women)
* live births per 1000 inhabitants (1988)   11,0
* population density per sq. kilometre (1987)   246
* minority groups: some, mainly from Mediterranean countries. Recent immigration from eastern European countries.

Health care system

Introduction   The Federal Republic of Germany is a federal state. At the Federal level the Ministry of 'Familie und Senioren' and the Ministry of Health are responsible for home care. Much power, however, is delegated to the federal states (Länder) and the various health insurance funds (Kranken-kassen) and there is no central planning for the whole of Germany. Instead, much is left to private initiative and governmental bodies only come into action if private initiative proves not to be able to reach minimal standards in health care. The states have the planning function related to hospitals.

Health insurance Germany forms an example of a pluralistic system of health insurance. In fact there are three options (figures taken from Crombie et al., 1990):

1   Public insurance (Gesetztliche Krankenkassenversicherung) through health insurance funds only: 85% of the population.
2   Public insurance supplemented by private insurance: 8% of the population.
3   Private insurance only: 7% of the population.

Public insurance is provided by a large number of health insurance funds (Krankenkassen) who are free to set their own level of contributions from employers and employees (within certain boundaries).

The GKV (Gesetzliche Krankenversicherung = Statutory Health Insurance) membership is compulsory for all workers and for all employees and for some categories of self-employees whose monthly income is below a certain amount of DM. The insured pay progressive contributions with the rate increasing with income.

Within the GKV a distinction is made between Pflichtkrankenkassen that insure mainly the blue collar workers and the Ersatzkrankenkassen for white collar workers. The local and regional Krankenkassen (health insurance funds) are the implementing bodies for the compulsory insurance. The health insurance funds are independent self-governing bodies with their own sovereignty and responsibility concerning the collection of contributions.

Funding

Table 5.1
Total expenditure on health care in the Federal Republic
of Germany (percent of GDP)

year	total expend. % GDP	public expend. % GDP	expend. in DM per head
1980	7.92	6.29	1902
1981	8.20	6.50	2048
1982	8.06	6.35	2093
1983	7.97	6.20	2176
1984	8.09	6.31	2327
1985	8.16	6.37	2449
1986	8.11	6.32	2563
1987	8.06	6.33	2642

Source: Program ECO-SANTE by CREDES and BASYS

Composition of total health care spending:
*   total expenditure on institutional health in % of total expenditure on health (1982, from OECD, 1985): 38.6
*   total expenditure on ambulatory health services in % of total expenditure on health (1982, from OECD, 1985): 26.7
*   total expenditure on pharmaceutics in % of total expenditure on health 1982), from OECD, 1985): 20.2.

Ambulatory care [4] Physicians strongly dominate German ambulatory care. These physicians are GPs as well as ambulatory specialists. There is free competition between all of them. The ambulatory physicians are self-employed. All ambulatory physicians are formally directly accessible. Patients have a free choice of doctor. Other health professionals often participate in ambulatory care as employees of a physician.

Only a GP or an independently practising specialist can refer a patient to a hospital.

According to Groenewegen et al. (1991) there are two types of General Practitioners: 'Allgemein Ärzte', specialists in general medicine, and 'Praktischer Ärzte' not specialised at all.

Single handed practice dominates, though a growing number of doctors participate in laboratory partnerships (several GPs using one laboratory) to profit from economies of scale.

In addition to consultation hours GPs often do home visits too.

GPs are remunerated on a fee for service basis by their professional organizations (Kassenärztliche Vereinigungen), which in turn receive their income from the Krankenkassen.

Patients are free to chose the GP they want, but once a choice is made, he is tied to it for the next 3 months. Patients are not registered with a GP.

In 1987 some 76,000 independent statutory health insurance physicians (1.1 per 1000 persons) practised in the Federal Republic, of which some 30,000 General Practitioners (Niedergelassene Allgemeinärzte). This means ± 0.5 GP per 1000 inhabitants.

Institutional care Ambulatory care and in-patient care are strictly divided. Hospitals dispense ambulatory care only on a limited scale and ambulatory physicians rarely treat their patients in hospitals.

There are two kinds of hospitals: hospitals for acute cases and special hospitals. The acute hospitals are meant for patients whose illness requires only a short hospital stay, while the special hospitals serve the chronically ill.

Table 5.2
In-patient medical care beds and personnel per bed

years	beds total	beds per 1000	personnel per bed
1980	707710	11.5	1.08
1981	695603	11.3	1.11
1982	683624	11.1	1.14
1983	682747	11.1	1.16
1984	678708	11.1	1.17
1985	674742	11.1	1.21
1986	674382	11.0	1.23
1987	673687	11.0	1.25

Source: Program ECO-SANTE by BASYS/CREDES

Community nursing

History Contemporary community nursing in Germany developed mainly from religious organizations. Almost every local community had a convent and community nursing care was usually delivered by nuns and 'diakonessen'. These religious organizations played an important role after the second world war in rebuilding the country. They were funded by the churches themselves and had nothing to do with insurance companies or other third party payment.

In the 1960s, however, the provision of home care was endangered by the fact that the religious became increasingly older and young people were not very much attracted by religious life. At the same time, it was realized that the growing elderly population would cause a greater need for home care in the near future. It was time for a major organizational change.

In mid-1970s the development of a network of 'Sozialstationen' began (Institut für Gerontologische Forschung, 1987), a new type of organization that took care of nursing for the ill and the elderly, and in some cases took care of the provision of home help services as well. The number of Sozialstationen continues to grow, but most areas seem to be covered now. According to a 1987 inventory study by the Deutscher Verein für öffentliche und private Fürsorge, 33% of all Sozialstationen offered not only community nursing services but also other types of care, in many cases home help care in 1984.

Organization After several experiments, a nationwide network of Sozialstationen developed, much of it still under the control of religious organizations. In 1984 there were between 1600 and 1900 of them (Institut für Gerontologische Forschung, 1987) with quite a lot of variation in their tasks, organization and personnel structure.

Although several Sozialstationen provide home help services and social work services as well, most of the Sozialstationen are primarily focused on home nursing of patients (Institut für Gerontologische Forschung, 1987). The reason for this lies in the fact that health insurance funds are the most important funding bodies. These health insurance funds, with some exceptions, only reimburse the costs of home nusring if this prevents patients from being hospitalized or if it is part of the medical treatment ordered by a general practitioner (ibid.).

In Germany there are six umbrella organizations for Sozialstationen:

1   Diakonisches Werk, which is an umbrella organization for Sozialstationen with a protestant background;
2   Caritas, which is an umbrella organization for Sozialstationen with a catholic background;
3   Arbeiterwohlfahrt, which is an umbrella organization for Sozialstationen with historical connections with the Social Democrat Party;
4   Deutsches Rotes Kreuz, the German Red Cross;
5   Deutscher Paritätischer Wohlfahrtsverband, an umbrella organization for independently organized Sozialstationen;
6   Zentralwohlfahrtsstelle der Juden in Deutschland, an umbrella organization for Jewish Sozialstationen.

The umbrella organizations maintain relations and negotiate with Krankenkassen and social insurance bodies to establish tariffs and to determine the tasks of Sozialstationen. In some cases, these umbrella organizations not only have a function towards Sozialstationen, but sometimes also towards homes for the elderly, hospitals and social services. Almost all Sozialstationen are non-profit organizations, but there are some for-profit and these are not part of the umbrella organizations mentioned above.

In urban regions there may be more than one Sozialstation in the area. In such cases people are free to choose the one they want. In some cases, however, there is a central office from which patients are referred. The number of Sozialstationen is small particularly in sparsely populated areas and people have to choose the one that is closest by.

In the Sozialstationen themselves there may be several types of personnel, including examinierte Krankenschwestern, examinierte Kinderkrankenschwestern, Altenpflegerinnen, Hauspflegerinnen, Familienpflegerinnen, and Sozialarbeiter. Nationwide there is a lot of variation between Sozialstationen in this respect. Furthermore, it is quite common that these Sozialstationen have volunteers helping them and 'Zivildienstleistenden', conscientious objectors to military service. An inventory in 1984 (Deutscher Verein für öffentliche und private Fürsorge, 1987) showed that 89% of the organizations offer nursing, 75% offer Altenpflege, and 49% offer Haus- und Familienpflege (see page 93 for descriptions of these types of care).

There are no formal regulations as to where a nurse can get specialist knowledge.

Generally speaking, child health care is not the task of Sozialstationen. In Berlin, however, and perhaps elsewhere too, there is a community nursing service for home care for children (Burmeister et al., 1989).

In normal cases healthy children are taken care of by the so-called Mutterberatung, a service that screens children and provides immunisations and which is provided by the local government, free of charge.

Some Sozialstationen have a 24-hour service.

Individual nurses may work on a solo basis or in a team. In one of the Sozialstationen that were visited each individual nurse took care of a single church community, a custom dating from the time when nurses were directly employed by these church communities. A team may consist of several types of nurses with sometimes social workers and home helps.

Funding Sozialstationen are funded by various bodies (Table 5.3).

Table 5.3
Sources of income of Sozialstationen (estimate)

federal or state taxes	10-20%
private insurance companies	<10%
public insurance companies	60%
patient out of pocket payment	10%
umbrella organizations	<10%

Source: questionnaire

State governments have stated criteria for Sozialstationen in order to receive funding. However, they are different for each member state. In general the amount of money paid by the government is dependent on the number and qualifications of personnel.

Patient fees are to be paid if:

1 The service received by a patient is not prescribed by a doctor.
2 The service received by a patient is prescribed by a doctor but not reimbursed by the public insurance company.

3   The service performed is not reimbursed by a private insurance company

4   A patient is not insured at all and the local social service does not want to pay.

5   The service is not reimbursed by an insurance company and the patient has too much income or capital for the social service to take over the costs.

Besides a block grant by the state, health insurance funds (Krankenkassen) are the most important financiers. Sozialstationen are reimbursed on a fee for service basis. In Berlin they are paid varying sums for a visit dependent on whether it concerns 'Grundpflege' or 'Behandlungspflege', insulin injections or 'Haushaltshilfe' (see page 93). Behandlungspflege is paid better than Grundpflege.

There are several conditions that have to be met. According to § 37 of the federal nursing law on 'häusliche Krankenpflege' home nursing and (to some extent) home help is reimbursed if:

1   hospitalization is necessary but not possible or can be shortened by home nursing or can be prevented

2   doctor's treatment needs to be combined with home nursing

3   family members can not take care of the patient themselves.

In any case home nursing should take place in combination with doctor's treatment. The maximum is three visits a day for four weeks. If it is necessary to continue after that, explicit approval is needed from the Krankenkassen

According to § 53 of the federal nursing law on Schwerpflegebedürftigen home nursing and home help are necessary and reimbursed if:

1   the patient, after assessment by a doctor, appears to be so helpless that he/she *chronically* needs *substantive* help with activities of daily living

2   and if the patient does not have rights according to § 37.

These patients are called Schwerpflegebedürftigen and they may receive 25 visits of 1 hour at most each month. The costs reimbursed by sick funds should not exceed DM 750 a month.

According to §57 of the federal nursing law, instead of receiving help with activities of daily living the patient may chose to organize his/her own home help and receive DM 400 from the Krankenkasse.

Both, § 53 and § 57, have been introduced on January 1 1991 and it is not yet possible to say anything about the consequences. According to a test-study by Brandt and Schweikart (1990) in Münster and Amberg two thirds of all Schwerpflegebedürftige would chose the DM 400.- and organize the home help care him/herself. According to more recent information (questionnaire) about 90% of all new applicants for home help care opt for the DM 400.--. Most of the new applicants seem not to have been cared for by Sozialstatione before.

Since 1989, informal carers who have cared for a Schwerpflegebedürftige for 12 months are allowed to take a four week vacation. During this vacation a professional nurse (this is called 'Urlaubspflege') can be employed, for which the Krankenkasse pays DM 1,800 to the patient. In 1989 there were 65,000 of these Urlaubspflege reimbursed by the Krankenkassen.

Home help care is reimbursed by most Krankenkassen and takes place if it is no longer possible to run a household without any professional help.

Sozialstationen are paid on a fee for service basis. During one of the authors' visits, a practical problem connected with this type of funding was encountered. Many patients receive more than one type of care during a visit. We were informed, however, that the number of services that are reimbursed for each visit is limited. In such a case the nurse chooses to write down only the most expensive ones.

The nurses themselves are paid a fixed monthly salary. They may also be paid on an hourly basis.

Recent developments A change in the funding system is currently under discussion in Germany. Though the various participants in this discussion have different plans, there is one common feature. The common feature is that all participants want to make the reimbursed sum dependent on the patient's level of dependency (Tophoven, 1991).

Types of community nurses and manpower

General In general four types of qualified nurses working in the community are discerned:
- Krankenschwester
- Kinderkrankenschwester
- Altenpflegerin
- Krankenpflegehelferin

Of these the Krankenschwester is a nurse generalist, while the Kinderkrankenschwester is specialized in the care for sick children and the Altenpflegerin is specialized in old people. The Krankenpflegehelferin represents the second level of expertise.

In addition to the nurses mentioned above, there are two types of personnel who are more home helps than nurses, though they do some nursing too:
- Hauspflegerin (home-help)
- Familienpflegerin (family help)

However, there is much variation among states concerning the work of Hauspflege/ Familienpflege. In some states there is no formal education, while in other states a two-year study does exist.

Education [5] The 1985 Federal Nursing Law (Krankenpflegegesetz) states the qualifications needed for the profession of 'Krankenpfleger/ Krankenschwes-

ter', 'Kinderkrankenschwester/Kinderkrankenpfleger' and 'Krankenpflege-
helferin/Krankenpflegehelfer'. Qualifications required for the profession of
Altenpflegerin/Altenpfleger are defined in the state laws (Landesgesetze).
Nursing schools should be attached to hospitals. Table 5.4 gives a summary of
nursing training in Germany. It should be remembered that in many states
schools for Familienpflege/ Hauspflege are absent. During one of the
author's visits, it appeared that much of the housekeeping work is being done
by people who are not formally trained for it.

Table 5.4
Basic nursing training in Germany

title	years of training	hours theoretical	hours on the job
Kranken-schwester	3 years	1600	3000
Kinderkranken-schwester	3 years	1600	3000
Altenpflegerin	2-3 years	1400-2240	1200-3000
Kranken-pflegehilfe	1 year	500	1100
Familien-pflege/ Hauspflege*	2 years	18 months	6 months

* formal training as Familienpflege/ Hauspflege exists only in some
  member states (Deutscher Verein für öffentliche und private Fürsorge,
  1987)

The practical parts of the various training schemes can take place in hospitals
or in any other organization, except for Krankenpflegehilfe where it only
takes place in nursing homes or hospitals.

There are several possibilities for further training. Specialization into
community nursing takes an other year (800 hours theoretical, 25 weeks on
the job) and can only be undertaken by (Kinder)krankenschwester after they
have worked for at least 2 years in that profession. A university program in
Nursing has recently been introduced.

Manpower Analogous to the organizational history of community nursing, with a decline of church related care during the sixties and seventies, the number of Gemeindekrankenschwester and -pfleger in Hessen declined from the mid-sixties (1966: 1310 persons) through 1977 (867 persons) and rose again to the 1966 level in 1983 (Deppe and Priester, 1987). This development seems to have taken place nationwide.

Furthermore, it has to be noted that there seems to be quite some local variation in manpower. Nurse-population ratios in the Mainz-Kinzig-Kreis in the state of Hessen in the mid-eighties varied from municipality to municipality between 288 and 2220 inhabitants per nurse. Twenty-one out of twenty-nine municipalities appeared to have less than one nurse per 3.500 inhabitants (Deppe and Priester, 1987) which is widely accepted as the best ratio.

In West-Berlin the number of inhabitants per nurse declined rapidly between 1984 and 1988 (Table 5.5)

Table 5.5
Number of inhabitants per community nurse in West-Berlin*

	all nurses**	'registered nurses'***
1984	1115	3255
1985	1188	3438
1986	988	2703
1987	1052	2316
1988	905	1690

* Nurses working in non-profit Sozialstationen only.
** Including examinierte Krankenschwestern, examinierte Kinderkrankenschwestern, Altenpflegerinnen, Hauspflegerinnen, Familienpflegerinnen, and Sozialarbeiter.
*** Including examinierte (Kinder)Krankenschwester only.

Source: calculated from Jahresgesundheitsbericht, 1988, Senatsverwaltung für Gesundheit und Soziales, 1990a)

The previously mentioned and generally accepted target figure of 3500 inhabitants per nurse is definitely exceeded in Berlin. This, however, is not at all indicative of the situation in Germany as a whole: already in 1984 Berlin had the highest nurse density (2 to 3 times as many as in other states, see Table 5.6), though this was mainly due to the large number of second level nurses (Deutscher Verein für öffentliche und private Fürsorge, 1987).

The rapid development indicated by the figures of Berlin should also serve as a warning not to make statements about the nurse-population ratio nowadays. If the nurse-density could double from 1984 to 1988 in Berlin one has to be very careful with the national figures from 1984 presented in Table 5.6.

Table 5.6
Number of nurses (full-time equivalents) per 10,000 inhabitants in German states in 1984

Schleswig-Holstein	4.6
Hamburg	5.3
Niedersachsen	4.1
Bremen	4.4
Nordrhein-Westfalen	2.8
Hessen	2.6
Rheinland-Pfalz	3.0
Baden-Württemberg	4.0
Bayern	3.0
Saarland	2.5
Berlin (west)	11.0
Bundesrepublik	**3.6**

Source: Deutscher Verein für öffentliche und private Fürsorge, 1987

According to the previously mentioned 1984 inventory study (Deutscher Verein für öffentliche und private Fürsorge, 1987) there were a total number of 36,354 people working in ambulatory services in the Federal Republic, accounting for 21,893 full-time equivalents (Table 5.7).

Table 5.7
Composition of total group of nursing personnel working in ambulatory care (n=21893), absolute number of full-time equivalents and number of inhabitants per nurse

	%	no. of full time equiv.	no. of inhabitants per nurse
Krankenschwester	47%	(10257)	5977
Altenpflegerin	9%	(1959)	31295
Haus- und Familienpflegerin/ Dorfhelferin	13%	(2972)	20628
Krankenpflegehelferin	6%	(1310)	46799
Helferin	25%	(5395)	11364
total	100%	(21893)	2800

Source: Deutscher Verein für öffentliche und private Fürsorge, 1987 and own computations

There was much variation between the states concerning the composition of personnel in Sozialstationen. For example in Hamburg only 10% were Krankenschwester and almost 80% were Helferin, whereas in Rheinland-Pfalz this was 60% and 8% respectively.

Patient populations According to several sources the size of the population that is being served by a Sozialstation varies between 12,000 and 50,000, also dependent on the size of the Sozialstation and degree of urbanization. Usually urban areas have a larger number of inhabitants per Sozialstation. Each memberstate has so called 'Förderrichtlinien' which sometimes state a range regarding the number of inhabitants that should be served by a Sozialstation.

Table 5.8
Characteristics of patients cared for by Sozialstationen

residence	age	patient category
- home	0-60 5-20%	- mainly chronically
- home for elderly (seldom)	> 60 80-95%	ill (about 90%)

Source: questionnaires

In Berlin 1986 there were 56 Sozialstationen. They had 6054 patients during one week in October (Senator für Gesundheit und Soziales, 1987).

According the previously mentioned study by Brandt and Schweikart (1990) about 50% of the Schwerpflegebedürftigen is above 80 years of age and about 85% is over 65. About 50% of them concerned illnesses of the central nerve system and 43% cerebrovascular illnesses. About 40% had both. Another large category was illnesses of the skeleto-muscular system with 26% of all cases.

Types of care

In community nursing, a very important - legal - distinction is made between 'Grundpflege' and 'Behandlungspflege'.

'Grundpflege' includes helping the patient with basic needs, including psychosocial activities; ADL activities; IADL activities; preventive care for instance for decubitus or pneumonia; checking and if necessary providing drinks and food; observation of for instance blood pressure or respiration; mobilization (Senatsverwaltung für Gesundheit und Soziales, 1990b).

'Behandlungspflege' includes the more technical nursing activities like injections, intravenous infusions, drip feeding, dressings, 'medical bath', oxygen therapy (Senatsverwaltung für Gesundheit und Soziales, 1990b).

In some cases the difference between Grundpflege and Behandlungspflege is not very clear (for instance rubbing ointment). This has consequences for reimbursement, since Behandlungspflege is better paid than Grundpflege and Sozialstationen may be tempted to regard certain activities as Behandlungspflege rather than Grundpflege and receive better payment.

The test-study by Brandt and Schweikart (1990) provides figures on the frequency of various types of care in Münster and Amberg. About 75% of the Schwerpflegebedürftigen was visited daily and about 20% weekly. Of those visited daily, about 25% received more than 1 visit a day.

About 67% received Grundpflege *and* Behandlungspflege and 13% received these types of care as well as home help care. Though no comparison is made with 'ordinary' patients of Sozialstationen, it is clear that Schwerpflegebedürftigen represent the most difficult cases.

The two types of nursing are in general carried out by Krankenschwestern, and with the exception of technical nursing procedures by Krankenschwesterhelferinnen and Altenpflegerinnen. Care like bathing and preparing medicine are sometimes done by Haus- or Familienpflegerinnen.

Home visits take about 80 to 90 percent of the total working time of these nurses. About 5% is spent on consultation hours and 5 to 10% on paperwork (qualified nurses more than auxiliaries). Very little time is spent on preventive home visits to elderly people (about 2%).

A third type of care is 'Haus- und Familienpflege/ Haushaltshilfe'. The

93

three names illustrate the confusion about what it is and by whom it should be done (see also section on Education). In Berlin it includes only urgent shopping and cleaning.

Stages in nursing

The previously mentioned study in Hessen (Deppe and Priester, 1987) mentions several possibilities for initiating nursing care:

- Patients living at home or their families or friends turn to a nurse or organization. The nurse cares for the patient independent of the physician. Only in case of necessary medical treatment the nurse turns to the physician.
- The nurse takes initiative to visit a patient without he or she having asked for it. Usually this too happens without notifying a physician. Possibilities to do this are very limited because of limited resources.
- Hospitals contact the Sozialstation a few days before the patient is discharged from hospital and the nurse consequently visits the patient at home.
- Most of the time, however, the general practitioner asks the Sozialstation to make an appointment with a patient and to carry out nursing activities.

Data on the percentage distribution of who initiates the first contact with the Sozialstation varies locally and educated guesses varied so much that one is hardly justified in making any general statement. The three most important initiators, however, appeared to be the general practitioner, hospital or nursing home, and the patient himself or his family.

Assessment is done either by a nurse, a head nurse or a physician. In almost all cases doctors orders are needed for reimbursement. The forms for assessment - used in some Sozialstationen - are in many cases adapted to this and state every item that can be reimbursed. The head nurse of the Sozialstation usually decides who is going to deliver the care. This is usually the nurse who is serving the particular area in which the patient lives.

In case of failures, physician are responsible for their orders and nurses are responsible for their own actions, further if she does not have the expertise to follow the doctor's orders, at least in Berlin. The head nurse is responsible for failures assigning a nurse to a patient and for failures during assessment. The employer is responsible for maintaining enough qualified personnel (Der Senator für Gesundheit und Soziales, 1987).

Relations with general practitioners, home help services and hospitals

General Practitioners Formally the nurse is dependent on doctor's orders. Only those activities are reimbursed by the Krankenkasse which are indicated by the doctor (which does not mean that everything that is ordered by a doctor is always reimbursed). However, in many cases the nurse visits a patient without doctor's orders and makes her own plan, asking the doctor for his permission afterwards (Deppe and Priester, 1987). Most nurses judge their relation with GPs as positive, though there are exceptions. This appeared from the study by Deppe and Priester as well as from the author's personal contacts with nurses. There is, however, a need for a more clear distinction between activities that should be reserved to doctors on the one hand and nurses on the other (Deppe and Priester, 1987). One of the items of discussion on this subject are infusions and applying intravenous injections with for example patients suffering from AIDS or cancer.

Contacts with general practitioners usually have an ad-hoc character.

In Berlin (in 1986) (Senator für Gesundheit und Soziales, 1987) most GPs (81%) cooperate with 1 to 3 Sozialstationen. A large number of doctors was aware of the services delivered by Sozialstationen, but only 27% knew all the services that were delivered in their working area. Most doctors (68%) deemed Sozialstation-personnel sufficiently qualified, but 37% thought there was too much unqualified personnel. It should be remembered that these figures are relatively old and that much may have been changed.

Home Help Services As we stated before, several Sozialstationen provide home help services as well as nursing services. These services are performed by 'Hauspflegerinnen' and 'Familienpflegerinnen'. There is some discussion about the division of tasks between nurses and home help personnel.

Hospitals Contacts with hospitals usually take place in case of aftercare needed by a patient. Friendships and occupational relations between individual persons play an important role and cooperation is usually organized informally. Contact by telephone is most usual but sometimes patients are visited in hospitals too (Deppe and Priester, 1987).

Though discharge and shortening the length of stay in hospitals is one of the major tasks of home care according to § 37 of the Federal Social Law there are no liaison nurses who are assigned to maintaining relations between Sozialstationen and hospitals and who deliver aftercare.

Other Sozialstationen The existence of more Sozialstationen in one area is usually not a problem (Deppe and Priester, 1987). A Sozialstation in the area of Frankfurt recently had started a central office from which patients would be assigned to specific Sozialstationen. Until then, however, contacts were infrequent and most of the times it concerned a request to another Sozialstation to take over a patient because of lack of time.

Problems

Underperformance According to experts the most underperformed tasks are those with elderly people. Though Sozialstationen are working almost exclusively for elderly people, this is apparently not enough. The problem mainly concerns psychosocial activities, encouragement of help by family members, provision of information on for instance medicine, health promotion in general and home help care. It has to be noted that the intensity of these problems varies locally.

Personnel shortages In many areas there is a shortage of community nurses, particularly qualified nurses (Krankenschwester). The generally accepted norm of 3,500 inhabitants per nurse would mean a need for 17,500 nurses nationwide. Instead there are about 10,000. Especially in southern Germany the need seems to be substantial (Brandt and Schweikhart, 1990).
Part of the problem is that many nurses stay in the profession only a few years. Reasons for this may be a shortage of opportunities for further education, conflicts with GPs (conflict between working independently and being dependent on doctor's orders) and unattractive aspects of the nursing profession in terms of income and in general work satisfaction. In addition, nurses in hospitals are paid better.
Waiting lists exist in some areas. If they do not exist, it does not mean that there is enough community nursing in an area. It is true that an organization is needed to make a waiting list. If there is no organization, there can not be a waiting list.

Specialist versus generalist No problems were reported on this issue.

Levels of experience and home helps Some problems were reported on the division of tasks between first and second level nurses.
As regards home helps, there is uncertainty on the required training of Haushaltshilfen and Familienpfleger, their tasks and responsibilities and how they relate to the tasks of Krankenpflegehelferinnen.

Community nursing and general practitioner Deppe and Priester (1987) complain about the fact that cooperation with general practitioners is weak and scarcely formalized. This in spite of the fact that the nurse is almost always dependent on referrals by general practitioners.
Deppe and Priester also mention the autonomy of nurses being hampererd by the fact that doctors orders are needed for all kinds of treatment.

Hospital and community nursing According to Deppe and Priester (1987) cooperation between community nurses and hospitals is hardly ever formalized and usually takes place on an ad-hoc basis.

Funding Deppe and Priester (1987) are in favor of a holistic approach in community nursing. However, they state that in the funding regulations a distinction is made between 'ill people', 'people who need nursing' and 'people who need help with activities of daily living'. This distinction is artificial since, in many cases the three types are united into one person.

Furthermore, reimbursement takes place on an item of service basis but these items do not include psychosocial activities. Most of the experts consulted in the study by Deppe and Priester are in favor of block grants instead of a fee for service system.

The system of reimbursement is currently under discussion and it is probable that a new system will be introduced in which the reimbursed sum varies with the patient's level of dependency.

Other problems Not all areas in Germany are equally covered by Sozialstationen yet. There are large regional differences.

According to Neuhaus and Schräder (1985), and Deppe and Priester (1987), there is a need for more centralized planning.

Brandt and Schweikart (1990) foresee problems in guarding the quality of care in cases where patients decide to opt for DM 400.- and organize the home help and Grundpflege themselves. They also pose the question as to what can be done to guard Sozialstationen from assigning less qualified personnel to Grundpflege in order to save money.

References

Brandt, F., R. Schweikart (1990), *Häusliche Pflegehilfen für Schwerpflegebedürftigen; Zwischenbericht zum Modellversuchs de Bundesministers für Arbeit und Sozialordnung*, Institut für Sozialforschung und Sozialwirtschaft e.V., Saarbrücken.

Burmeister, I., N. Goschin, E. Holthaus, J. Korporal, H. Müller, J. Räbiger, U. Rahe-Badenhoop, H. Wilke, A. Zink (1989), *Häusliche Kinderkrankenpflege; Modellprojekt externer Pflegedienst in Berlin, Band II: Ergebnisse der sozialmedizinischen und ökonomische Begleitung*, Robert Bosch Stiftung, Bleicher Verlag, Gerlingen.

Crombie, D.L., P. Backer, J. Van Der Zee (eds.) (1990), *The Interface Study: COMAC-HSR in collaboration with European General Practice Research Workshop*, RCGP, London.

Deppe, H-U., K. Priester (1987), Modelluntersuchung Ambulante Krankenpflege; Arbeitsweise und Stellung im Gesundheitswesen, HLT Gesellschaft für Forschung Planung Entwicklung mbH, Wiebaden.

Der Senator für Gesundheit und Soziales (1987), *Die Berliner Sozialstationen: Angebot und Entwicklung*, Bearbeitet von Priv.-Doz. Dr. G. Meinlschmidt und Marlies Wanjura, Berlin.

Deutscher Verein für öffentliche und private Fürsorge (1987), *Bestandsaufnahme der ambulanten sozialpflegerischen Dienste (Kranken- und Altenpflege, Haus- und Familienpflege) im Bundesgebiet*, Bearbeitet von R. Höft-Dzemski, Band 65 Schriftenreihe des Bundesministers für Jungend, Familie, Frauen und Gesundheit, W. Kohlhammer GmbH, Stuttgart.

Groenewegen, P.P., J. Van Der Zee, R. Van Haaften (1991), *Remunerating General Practitioners in Western Europe*, Avebury, Aldershot.

Institut für gerontologische Forschung (1987), *Gutachten über Sozialstationen*, München.

Landesversorgungsamt Bayern (1989), *Richtlinien zur Förderung ambulanter sozialpflegerischer Dienste*, München.

Neuhaus, R., W.F. Schräder (1985), Planning and management of public health in the Federal Republic of Germany, *Health Policy*, 5, pp. 99-109.

OECD (1988), *Ageing populations; the social policy implications*, Organisation for economic co-operation and development, Paris.

OECD (1985), *Measuring health care 1960-1983; expenditure, Costs and Performance*, Organisation for economic co-operation and development, Paris.

Schnell, W (1987), *Krankenpflegegesetz mit Ausbildungs- und Prüfungsverordnung: Handbuch zur Aus- und Weiterbildung in der Krankenpflege*, Reha-Verlag, Bonn.

Senatsverwaltung für Gesundheit und Soziales (1990a), *Jahresgesundheitsbericht 1988*, Berlin.

Senatsverwaltung für Gesundheit und Soziales (1990b), 'Rundschreiben über Abschluß einer neuen Entgelvereinbarung über Hausliche Krankenpflege, Haushaltshilfe und häusliche Pflege für Schwangere', In: *Ambtsblatt für Berlin* 40, 55, 2 November.

Statistical yearbook of Norway 1990 (1990), Statistisk Sentralbyrå, Oslo-Kongsvinger.

Tophoven, L (1991), *Die Absicherung des Pflegerisikos aus Sichte der GKV*, In: Arbeit und Sozialpolitik pp. 3-4.

Notes

1. Co-author of this paragraph is drs. Paul van der Heijden.

2. Sources:
   - M. Schneider et al (1989), *Gesundheitssysteme im internationalen Vergleich: laufende Berichterstattung für den Bundesminister für Arbeit und Sozialordnung*, BASYS, Augsburg.
   - B. Abel-Smith, *Eurocare: European health care analysis*, HeathEcon s.a., Basle.
   - E. Carrillo et al (1989), *Requirements & constraints for minimum data sets*, McAce, S.L.
   - D.L. Crombie et al (1990), *The interface study*, The Royal College of General Practitioners, London.
   - Federal minister for youth, family affairs, women and health (1988), *The health care system in the Federal Republic of Germany*, Schmidt & Klaunig, Kiel.

3. Sources: Statistical Yearbook of Norway (1990); OECD (1988).

4. Sources: Crombie et al (1989); Groenewegen et al (1991).

5. Main source: Schnell (1987).

6 Community nursing in the Netherlands

The setting [1]

Population [2]
* total population (1987)   14,7 million
* % over 65 (1988)   12,5
* % over 65 (2000, projected)   13,5
* % over 65 (2010, projected)   15,1
* % over 65 (2020, projected)   18,9
* % under 15 (1988)   18,5
* life expectancy at birth (years)(1987)   73,4 (men)
                                                  79,9 (women)
* live births per 1000 inhabitants   12,6
* population density per sq. kilometre (1987)   359
* population groups: immigration in the '60s, '70s and '80s from Mediterranean countries and Suriname.

Health care system

Introduction   The Netherlands is a constitutional monarchy. Very little political power is delegated to the provincial and local levels.

Overall responsibility for statutory health insurance rests with the Minister of Welfare, Health and Cultural affairs (Ministerie van Welzijn, Volksgezondheid en Cultuur). The final decision regarding planning, charges, benefits and contribution rates rests with the Minister. The Health Inspectorate attached to the ministry supervises and monitors the standards of health care. In one of the most recent publications (WVC, 1991a) a future shift of responsibilities from the central government to professional care givers, health insurance funds and patients.

The National Health Council gives advice about planning, structure, provision, quality and efficiency of health care in general, and on the implementation of the two health insurance schemes.

The planning of hospital construction lies with the Board for Hospital Facilities.

The Central Health Charges Board is responsible for approving and laying down health service tariffs and establishes guidelines concerning the level, structure and method of calculation.

The Health Insurance Fund Council advises the ministry on the administration and planning of statutory health insurance and on managing the funds.

Health insurance [3] The health insurance system can be divided into two schemes:

- A compulsory health insurance scheme for all employees below a fixed wage level, old age pensioners who were publicly insured prior to retirement, and persons in receipt of social benefits. In 1987 this insurance covered 61.5% of the population.
- The rest of the population have to insure themselves against the cost of illness by private insurance. Privately insured persons have a range of options with varying coverage and co-payments, deductibles and so on.

Insurance for exceptional medical expenses is covered by the Exceptional Medical Expenses Act (Algemene Wet Bijzondere Ziektekosten), which applies to all residents of the Netherlands without any restrictions. This supplementary scheme started as a cover for 'heavy risks' not provided for under the health insurance scheme (stay in hospitals for over a year and stay in nursing homes and institutions for the mentally retarded from the first day), but is now gradually being extended to community nursing (1980), ambulatory mental health care (1985), all mental health care and home help (1989), and medical appliances (1990).

Plans for a comprehensive basic insurance system are in an advanced stage of development. All basic services, defined in terms of functions will be covered by this insurance. This new system will have to be implemented by insurance companies. In addition to the basic functions, insurance companies will be able to provide possibilities for additional insurance (WVC, 1991a).

In the plans for this new basic insurance scheme (WVC, 1991a) the suggestion is made that professional home care should only be provided where informal care does not suffice.

Funding The compulsory scheme is mainly financed by contributions of employees and employers. Deficits are subsidized by the government. The scheme is administered by approximately forty autonomous health insurance funds operating on a regional basis under supervision of the Health Insurance Fund Council (Ziekenfondsraad), an independent body that also advises

102

on the contribution and premium levels, which are the same nationwide.

Private insurance is paid by premiums of the insured. The privately insured have a range of options with varying coverage and co-payments, deductibles and so on.

The general scheme against high risk (Act on Exceptional Medical Expenses) is funded by general taxation.

Table 6.1
Expenditure on health care in the Netherlands

year	total expen. % GDP	public expen. % GDP	expend. in DFL per head
1980	8.19	6.21	1949
1981	8.38	6.38	2076
1982	8.58	6.58	2206
1983	8.61	6.57	2279
1984	8.33	6.38	2308
1985	8.22	6.26	2365
1986	8.31	6.11	2445
1987	8.46	6.25	2484

Source: Program ECO-SANTE by CREDES and BASYS

As the table shows, the expenditure on health care as a percentage of the GDP remains fairly stable, although the expenditure in DFL per head increases. In comparison with other OECD countries however the percentages spent on health care are one of the highest.

Ambulatory care [4] General practitioners function as 'gatekeepers' of the health care system. A patient has to consult a GP before consulting a medical specialist. The GP therefore determines access to other parts of the health care system and is the point of referral. For publicly insured patients the referral is mandatory. Private insurance carriers usually also require a referral. The GP is usually an independent entrepreneur. Most of them work alone but an increasing number are engaged in group practice and in multi-professional teams in health centres.

GPs receive a capitation fee for each publicly insured patient on their list, a full tariff for the first 1,600 patients and a lower tariff for the rest. Fees are paid periodically to the GPs by the health insurance funds. GPs are paid on a fee-for-service basis by privately insured patients or their insurance companies. Practically every GP has both publicly and privately insured patients. However, the actual balance differs according to the prosperity of the community.

In 1987 there were 6,243 general practitioners in the Netherlands (Centraal Bureau voor de Statistiek, 1989).

Ambulatory specialist care is only provided (after referral) by the outpatient departments of hospitals. Specialists do not work in the community.

Institutional Care [5] Most of the hospitals in the Netherlands are privately owned hospitals and they all are non-profit organizations. The gGovernment has an important say in hospital funding. The hospital system is well developed, comprising a network of general, single-specialty and university hospitals. General (acute) hospitals provide the entire range of basic-specialties of medicine, surgery and obstetric care. Between these three types of hospitals no hierarchical relations exist. All general hospitals provide outpatient care, and long stay hospitals are developing day care centres.

Table 6.2
Inpatient medical care beds and personnel per bed

year	beds total	beds per 1000	personnel per bed
1980	127481	9.0	1.43
1981	127206	8.9	1.45
1982	124039	8.6	1.52
1983	123736	8.6	1.50
1984	123522	8.5	1.51
1985	123320	8.5	1.51
1986	122702	8.4	1.54
1987	122353	8.3	1.55

Source: Program ECO-SANTE by CREDES and BASYS

Most specialists operate from private practices at the outpatient departments of hospitals.

In the 1980s the total number of beds declined with some 5,000 beds. The number of beds per 1000 inhabitants declined with 0.7 bed and the personnel per bed rose from 1.43 to 1.55 persons per bed.

Community nursing

Community nursing services as we defined them in the introduction are provided by a number of organizations which operate nationwide but which do not have the same tasks in every region:
- public health services: communicable disease control; environmental health screening of children between 4 and 19 years of age;
- occupational health services;
- ambulatory mental health care;
- a small number of for-profit nursing agencies;
- cross associations (see below).

In all these organizations various types of nurses are employed, who work in the community. In terms of numbers of nursing personnel, however, the cross associations are the most important.

Within the cross associations an organizational distinction is made between a division that provides community nursing care (preventive as well as curative care delivered by nurses) and a division that provides maternity home care. Maternity home care in the Netherlands consists of (Hingstman, 1991):
- assisting GP or midwife during delivery;
- physical care with the baby;
- helping with breast feeding;
- providing general health information;
- looking after family members and some housework.

This care is delivered during the first 8 days after delivery.

In the following we will concentrate on the preventive and curative services delivered by community nurses in regional cross associations.

History

In 1875, ten local community nursing organizations were established. The tasks of these 'Cross Associations', as they were called, was to combat epidemic diseases and to protect the population from the spread of diseases by disinfecting clothes, furniture and houses. They also lent material like beds and blankets to their members (Kerkstra, 1989).

Several organizational changes have taken place in the last decades. In the early 80s there was a shift in governmental policy from specialist and residential care towards home care and primary health care. As a consequence, from 1980 to 1986 the budget of the cross associations was allowed to grow by 4% each year. From 1986 onwards the allowable increase was fixed at 2%. This policy has had some impact on the quantitative development of community nursing manpower. However, in 1988, the budget was reduced again (Kerkstra, 1989).

From 1980 onwards, a compulsory public insurance scheme based on the

105

General Act on Exceptional Medical Costs (AWBZ), made it possible for everyone to obtain community nursing care.

Since 1989, a large reorganization has been taking place. The number of regional cross associations has been reduced from 160 in 1987 to 70 in 1990. In the new situation a regional cross association has a catchment area of approximately 230.000 inhabitants.

In 1990 the umbrella organizations for community nursing (National Cross Association) and for home help services were integrated into the National Association for Home Care. During the next five years, this integration is also going to take place at the level of regional cross associations.

It is expected that this integration will increase the efficiency in home care and will avoid unnecessary overlap between community nursing and home help services (WVC, 1990).

Organization and funding

Organization Dutch community nursing care is organized at different levels, as you can see below.

National Association for Home Care

± 70 Regional Cross Associations (estimate)

± 500 Basic Units (estimate)

The National Association for Home Care is an umbrella organization and has four main duties: to prepare policy on the national level, to promote the interests of its members, to engage in collective bargaining with government and insurance companies, and to provide services to the regional cross associations (Landelijke Vereniging voor Thuiszorg, 1991).

The regional organizations consist of a number of basic units. In these basic units, a chief nursing officer (head nurse), about ten community nurses and two or three auxiliary nurses work in a team. Due to continuing reorganizations the exact number of regional cross associations and basic units could not be determined.

Two levels of expertise are employed by the regional cross associations and a number of dieticians and child health clinic physicians. Specialist knowledge is provided by so called 'nurse specialists'. They are usually not concerned with direct patient care and are employed by regional cross associations. The nurse specialists can be consulted by regular nurses concerning concrete patient situations. They also have a supporting role in the development of special care programs (Verbeek, 1991).

Nurses work in basic units, consisting of about 11 nurses (including a head nurse), and 2 auxiliaries. A basic unit is assigned to a defined geographical area (about 35.000 inhabitants). Within this team each individual nurse, or a sub-team of a few nurses and an auxiliary, is assigned to a specific sub-area (Vorst-Thijssen et al, 1990).

Cross associations can be reached 24 hours a day and care can be delivered in the evenings, nights and weekends if necessary.

Patients are entitled to a maximum amount of care: 2.5 hours a day or 3 visits a day, for an unlimited period of time. There are associations for patients with terminal illness for additional home care for a limited period of time.

Funding Since 1980 the cross associations are funded for about 85 % through a system of public insurance based on the General Act on Exceptional Medical Costs (AWBZ)(Ministerie van Welzijn, Volksgezondheid en Cul-´ tuur, 1990). Under the provisions of this Act, all residents of the Netherlands are entitled to community nursing care and no prescription from a physician is needed except for medical treatment. Regional cross associations receive a fixed amount of money from AWBZ, based on the number of personnel. Taxes are raised by the central government.

The remaining 15% is largely paid from patient's membership fees which vary regionally (average Dfl. 50 each year per family). This annual fee can be regarded as co-payment. There are no specific services and/or interventions for which out of pocket payment is necessary. The regional cross associations are free to determine the level of the membership fees within certain limits. Cross associations with higher membership fees can provide extra care or service facilities.

There are minimal standards that have to be met by the cross associations in order to be funded by the state:

Types of care: (1) nursing activities in the home related to illness, disability, old age; (2) care for mother and child, including periodic assessment of the child's health; (3) providing equipment in loan; (4) activities directed at prevention of illness and unhealthy habits.

Accessability: 24 hours a day, in order to be able to provide care in urgent cases.

Manpower in direct patient care:

1 community nurse for every 3450 inhabitants.

1 auxiliary nurse for every 3 community nurses.

1 head nurse for every 9 community nurses and/or auxiliary nurses. This standard, however, has become obsolete.

Quality control: state enrolled inspectors of public health have to be admitted free access at all times.

(Erkenningsnormen Kruisorganisaties, 1981).

Nurses receive a fixed monthly salary.

Types of community nurses and manpower

Education There are four types of community nurses employed by the cross associations:
'Wijkverpleegkundigen' (community nurses) who have had either 4 years of higher vocational training or 3½ years in-service training with 2 years of intermediate vocational training.
'Wijkziekenverzorgenden' (auxiliary community nurses) who either have had 2 years in-service training in hospital or nursing home for the elderly and a 6-month course in community nursing or 3 years intermediate vocational training in nursing. (Source: Adriaanse and Van der Laan, 1989)
'Wijkverpleegkundigen' can become head nurses after having worked for at least two years in community nursing. One has to follow a 2-year course of one day a week.

To become a nurse specialist, it is possible to follow an 18th month course and graduate in either professional innovation, management or as a clinical nurse specialist. One can graduate as a clinical nurse specialist in elderly care, child health care or chronic health problems (among which diabetes, oncology and rheumatoid arthritis).

There is also a 24 month masters degree in nursing at three universities with main subjects in clinical nursing, management and teaching.

Manpower [6] As the focus of government policy shifted from hospital care to community care the budgets for community care were allowed to grow considerably. This is reflected in a growing number of community nurses (and a decreasing nurse-population rate which is shown in Table 6.3). The table shows a larger increase in the number of second level nurses than in first level nurses.

Table 6.3
Number of inhabitants per community nurse and per auxiliary nurse
in the Netherlands 1982-1987

1982	3,219	inhabitants per community nurse
1983	3,156	(full-time equivalents)
1984	3,098	
1985	3,025	
1986	2,951	
1987	2,903	

1982	15,015	inhabitants per auxiliary nurse
1983	13,814	(full-time equivalents)
1984	12,690	
1985	12,210	
1986	11,655	
1987	11,327	

Source: CBS 1984, 1985, 1986, 1987, 1988, 1989

It can be seen in the table that there are more first level than second level nurses. In fact there are about 4 first level nurses for every second level nurse.

In addition to these types of nurses there were 162 child health clinic physicians, 188 dieticians, 527 head nurses and 241 nurse specialists employed by the cross associations in 1987 (Centraal Bureau voor de Statistiek, 1989).

Patient populations

According to government standards there should be one community nurse for every 3450 inhabitants, one auxiliary nurse for every three community nurses and 1 head nurse for every nine community nurses and/or community nurses (Besluit Erkenningsnormen, 1981). In 1983 the government indicated the desirable ratio was 1 community nurse for every 2500 inhabitants (WVC, 1983) and 3 community nurses for every auxiliary by the year 1990.
Figures in Table 6.3 show that this target had not yet been reached in 1987.

According to statistics of the National Cross Association (1986) 8.65% of the population received community nursing care.

Table 6.4 shows the age-distribution of patients receiving home visits. More than 85% of the patients are over 60. Home visits are paid to patients living in their own home as well as in elderly people's homes without comprehensive nursing services.

The small percentage of under 5s is due to the fact that most care for this category takes place during consultation hours and not during home visits. About 94% of the children under 1 pay visits to these child health clinic and 83% of all children between 1 and 4 (Centraal Bureau voor de Statistiek, 1985).

Table 6.4
Age distribution of patients receiving home visits by
regional cross associations

under 5's	0.3%
age 5 - 19	0.8%
age 20 - 59	12.4%
age 60 - 79	45.4%
80 and over	41.1%

Source: Vorst-Thijssen et al., 1990

One of the reasons for 68% of all home visits is some kind of disease. The distribution of these diseases is shown in Table 6.5.

Table 6.5
Diagnoses of patients receiving nursing care at home (n = 3315)

diagnosis	percentage
musculoskeletal disorders	27.1%
cardiovascular diseases	17.2%
diabetes	14.9%
no diagnosis (frailty, old age)	13.5%
cancer	12.6%
neurological disorders	12.2%
cerebral haemorrhage	9.6%
dementia senilis	6.6%
chronic obstructive pulmonary diseases	6.1%
other diagnosis	18.6%

Source: Vorst-Thijssen et al., 1990

The nurses work as generalists and care for all patient categories. It is questioned by many whether this situation should continue. According to Kerkstra (1991) the growing complexity and workload of curative tasks negatively affects the viability of working as a generalist.

Auxiliary nurses are generally speaking not concerned with child health care.

Types of care

Mother and child care usually takes place in child health clinic sessions in most cases with a physician. Care for the elderly takes place during home visits. The percentages of total working time spent on selected activities is shown in Table 6.6.

Table 6.6
Percentage of working time spent on selected activities by community nurses (N=108) and auxiliary nurses (N=49)

	nurses	auxiliaries
assessment visits	1.4%	0.6%
curative home visits	33.6%	49.6%
preventive home visits	6.0%	1.1%
child health clinic sessions	10.6%	2.5%
consultation hours	5.4%	4.5%
meetings	18.0%	18.8%
other, incl. paper work	15.7%	13.2%

Source: Vorst-Thijssen et al, 1990

Auxiliaries appear to be more concerned with home visits and less with paperwork than nurses. Nurses are responsible for child health clinic sessions, sometimes assisted by an auxiliary.

Table 6.7 shows the distribution of activities during home visits by nurses and auxiliaries. There appears only to be a significant difference between nurses and auxiliaries concerning hygienic care and support with psychosocial problems. The division of tasks is currently under discussion.

Table 6.7
Distribution of home visits according to type of care for
nurses and auxiliaries

	nurses	auxiliaries
personal hygienic care	58.7%	67.8%
technical nursing care	67.9%	70.4%
housework	24.4%	29.5%
health education	36.9%	35.7%
support with therapy	28.1%	24.5%
support psychosocial problems	34.7%	25.5%
support informal care	30.1%	28.9%
observation	20.0%	15.3%
social and adm. activities	65.9%	66.3%
total percentage*	366.7%	364.0%
total number of visits	5689	3512

*   more than one type of care can be delivered during a home visit

Source: Vorst-Thijssen et al., 1990

Table 6.8 gives the motives for home visits. Most of the care appears to be related to diagnosis (see also Table 6.5).

Table 6.8
Motives for visiting the patient at home (n = 3315)

motives*	percentage
terminal care	3.2
aftercare	5.7
patient education	4.8
reassurance	10.3
support in psychosocial problems	6.8
care related to diagnosis	67.6
hygienic care activities	27.5
other motives	6.6

*   28% of the home visits had more than one motive.

Source: Kerkstra and Vorst-Thijssen, 1991

Vorst-Thijssen et al. (1990) provide information on initiators of first contacts with cross organizations (Table 6.9).

Table 6.9
Percentage of patients noting by whom the first contact is initiated:

patient self/family	47%
general Practitioner	17%
home help service	2%
hospital or nursing home	34%
other	7%

Source: Vorst-Thijssen et al., 1990

Most patients appear to initiate the contact themselves, followed by those who are referred by hospitals or nursing homes.

Assessment is carried out by first level nurses, using standard forms in some regions. The decision as to who is going to deliver the care is taken by the same nurse, in co-operation with the head nurse. Generally speaking, the more complex cases are assigned to nurses and to auxiliaries in cases in which no difficult technical nursing care is to be delivered. As we saw earlier, however, the difference between nurses and auxiliaries is not very big if we look at activities during home visits. Nurses and auxiliaries are responsible for their own actions.

Evaluation takes place regularly in each basic unit, but the frequency varies.

Relations with general practitioners, home help services and hospitals

Consultation with General Practitioners takes place 3 to 4 times a month. Usually the contact concerns individual patients and takes place on an ad-hoc basis. The number of GPs an individual nurse has to deal with may vary from one in very rural areas to 70 in large cities (De Bakker, 1988). Discussion on the division of tasks between nurses and GPs concerning medical-technical activities has recently resulted in a law on Professions in Individual health care (Beroepen Individuele Gezondheidszorg).

Contacts with home help services are less frequent: 2 to 3 times a month (Vorst-Thijssen e.a., 1990). Usually these contacts too take place on an ad-hoc basis, though there are many examples of regular plenary meetings in which a number of patients is discussed. In the near future more and more home help agencies and community nursing services will integrate at the local level as is already the case now at the national level. In some cross associations assessment is already combined for home help and community nursing service. But in many cases the division of tasks between auxiliaries and home helps is problematic.

There are some examples of community based liaison nurses, so-called continuity nurses, who are especially assigned to maintaining relations with other care providers and safeguarding continuity of care (Kersten and Hackenitz, 1991).

Problems

Underperformance Information from the field learns that time is often lacking for psychosocial and preventive activities.

Personnel shortages In the Werner-report (WVC, 1991b) by the year 2000 a shortage of nursing personnel of 20% is predicted. Reasons for this shortage are:
- high workload
- student drop-out rate
- increasing number of part-timers
- lack of a clear division of tasks, because of which nursing personnel also sometimes have to do housework
- high level of absenteeism
- lack of career opportunity.

Specialist versus generalist The increasing workload and the growing complexity of care make a generalist method of working increasingly viable. In the study by Vorst-Thijssen et al. (1990), 46% of all community nurses appeared to be in favour of a more differentiated method of working (see also Buijssen and Burgers, 1990; and Ropping, 1989). In many cross associations discussion continues on this dilemma.

Levels of expertise and home helps Home help and community nursing are going to merge into one organization. A more efficient use of capacities is expected to result from this development. However, to reach this goal, it will be necessary to make the division of tasks between home helps and auxiliary nurses, and nurses and auxiliaries more clear.

Another question that arises is how and by whom the assessment should be carried out.

Community nursing and general practitioner The increasing options for technically advanced nursing at home raise the question as to what extent the nurse is liable to carry out this type of nursing. The division of tasks between nurses and general practitioners should be made more clear. The same is

114

true for the nurse's authority in prescription. In practice it happens often that a prescription by a general practitioner is obtained afterwards.

Suggestions in this respect are made in the report on Medical Interventions by the National Cross Association (the precursor of the National Association for Home Care) and the National General Practitioner's Association (Nationale Kruisvereniging en Landelijke Huisartsenvereniging, 1990).

Hospital and community nursing In many cases the communication between hospitals and cross associations could be improved. Wiegers and Kersten (1990) found that the problems mainly concern the preparations for discharge and time-continuity between hospital care and home care.

Funding The most important issue concerns the proposed changes in the health care system. In the proposed system cross associations may lose their monopoly and have to compete with other organizations in home care. In this system each cross association will have to contract with health insurance companies, and direct government funding will become absolute.

References

Adriaansen, M., B. Van Der Laan (1989), *Extramurale Gezondheidszorg; Functie en taken van de wijkverpleegkundige* [Community care; Function and tasks of the community nurse], Van Loghum Slaterus, Deventer.

Bakker, D.H. De (1988), *Afstemming van werkgebieden en doelpopulaties in de eerstelijns(gezonheids)zorg* [Attuning working area's and target populations in primary (health) care], NIVEL, Utrecht.

Besluit Erkenningsnormen Kruisorganisaties 1981 (1981), [Decree on recognition of cross associations], In: *MGZ*, 9, 7/8, juli/augustus, pp. 52-58.

Buijssen, H., N. Burgers (1988), 'Gedifferentieerd werken biedt voordelen, maar all-round werken blijft ideaal' [Specialist approach has advantages, but generalist approach still ideal], *Maatschappelijk Gezondheidszorg*, 16, 2, pp. 12-14.

Centraal Bureau voor de Statistiek (1989), *Vademecum Gezondheidsstatistiek Nederland* [Health Statistics], SDU, Den Haag.

Centraal Bureau voor de Statistiek (1984, 1985, 1986, 1987, 1988, 1989), *Maandbericht Gezondheidsstatistiek* [Health Statistics], Staatsuitgeverij, 's-Gravenhage.

Gloerich, A.B.M., R.T.J. Hamers, J. Van Der Zee, P.P. Groenewegen (1989) *Regional Variation in hospital admission rates in the Netherlands, Belgium and the North of France, Basic information and references*, Netherlands institute of primary health care, Utrecht.

Hingstman, L (1991), 'Primary care obstetrics and perinatal health in the Netherlands', Paper submitted to the *British Journal of Obstetrics and Gynaecology*, NIVEL, Utrecht.

Kerkstra, A. (1989), *Community nursing in the Netherlands*, In: A. Kerkstra & R. Verheij (eds.), Community Nursing, Proceedings of the International conference on community nursing, 16-17 March 1989, 's-Hertogenbosch, the Netherlands, Netherlands institute of primary health care, Utrecht.

Kerkstra, A (1991), Lessen uit het buitenland [Lessons from abroad], *Maatschappelijke Gezondheidszorg*, 19, 2, pp. 24-28.

Kerkstra, A. and T. Vorst-Thijssen (1991), 'Factors related to the use of community nursing services in the Netherlands', *Journal of Advanced Nursing*, 16, pp. 47-54.

Kersten, T.J.J.M.T. and E. Hackenitz (1991), 'How to bridge the gap between hospital and home', *Journal of Advanced Nursing*, 16, pp. 4-14.

Landelijke Vereniging voor Thuiszorg (1991), *Informationbrochure*, Landelijke Vereniging voor Thuiszorg, Bunnik.

Nationale Kruisvereniging (1989), *Jaarrapportage jeugdgezondheidszorg 0 - schoolgaand, Kruiswerk 1987* [Year report child health care], Nationale Kruisvereniging, Bunnik.

Nationale Kruisvereniging (1986), *Kruiswerk in Beeld* [Community nursing in the picture], Nationale Kruisvereniging, Bunnik.

Nationale Kruisvereniging en Landelijke Huisartsen Vereniging (1990), *Medisch handelen door verpleegkundige beroepsbeoefenaars in de thuissituatie*, [Medical treatment by nurses at home], deel 1, Nationale Kruisvereniging, Bunnik.

OECD (1988), *Ageing populations; the social policy implications*, Organization for economic co-operation and development, Paris.

Ropping, R. (1989), 'Haags Kruiswerk: speciale taken voor de wijkverpleging, maar iedereen wel in de patiëntenzorg' [Community nursing in The Hague: special tasks for nurses, but everyone wants to work with patients], *Maatschappelijke Gezondheidszorg*, 17, 11, pp. 12-14.

Statistical yearbook of Norway 1990 (1990), Statistisk Sentralbyrå, Oslo-Kongsvinger.

Verbeek, R. (1991), 'Wat doet de districtsverpleegkundige na de reorganisatie' [What will be the tasks of nurse specialist after the reorganization?], *Maatschappelijke Gezondheidszorg*, 19, 2, pp. 19-22.

Vorst-Thijssen, T. (1987), *De zorg voor zuigelingen en kleuters* [The care for infants and pre-school children], NIVEL, Utrecht.

Vorst-Thijssen, A., A. v.d. Brink-Muinen, A. Kerkstra (1990), *Het werk van wijkverpleegkundigen en wijkziekenverzorgenden in Nederland* [The work of wijkverpleegkundigen and wijkziekenverzorgenden in the Netherlands], NIVEL, Utrecht.

Wiegers, T.A., T.J.J.M.T. Kersten (1990), 'Problemen bij de overdracht van nazorgpatiënten: continuïteit onderzocht' [Problems in the transfer of patients needing aftercare: continuity investigated], *Tijdschrift voor Ziekenverpleging*, 22, pp. 728-732.

WVC (1990), *Heroverwegingsonderzoek, Van Samenwerken naar Samengaan. Gezinsverzorging en Kruiswerk naar een geïntegreerd aanbod in de thuiszorg. Rapport van de heroverwegingswerkgroep. Doelmatigheidsonderzoek organisatiestructuur gezinsverzorging en kruiswerk* [From collaboration to integration. Home help and community nursing towards integrated home care. Study on the efficiency of the organizational structure of home help services and community nursing], Ministerie van Welzijn, Volksgezondheid en Cultuur, Rijswijk.

WVC (1991a), *Thuiszorg aan bod: beleidsnotitie thuiszorg* [Home care at stake: policy document on home care], Ministerie van Welzijn, Volksgezondheid en Cultuur, Rijswijk.

WVC (1991b), *In hoger beroep: perspectief voor de verplegende en verzorgende beroepen* [Perspective for nurses and carers], Rapport van de Commissie Positiebepaling Beroep van Verpleegkundige en Verzorgende, Ministerie van Welzijn, Volksgezondheid en Cultuur, Rijswijk.

Notes

1. Co-author of this paragraph is drs. Paul van der Heijden.

2. Sources: Statistical Yearbook of Norway (1990); OECD (1988).

3. Main source: Groenewegen, P.P. et al (1991), *Remunerating General Practitioners in Western Europe*. Gower, Aldershot, p. 92-93.

4. Main source: Carrillo, E. et al (1989), *Requirements & constraints for minimum data sets*, McACE, S.L., p. 61.

5. Main source: Gloerich et al (1989).

6. Main source: CBS (1988).

7 Community nursing in Norway

The setting

Population
* total population (1987)   4,2 million
* % over 65 (1989)   16,2
* % over 65 (2000, projected)   15,2
* % over 65 (2010, projected)   15,1
* % over 65 (2020, projected)   18,2
* % under 15 (1989)   18,9
* life expectancy at birth (years) (1988)   73,1 (men)
     79,6 (women)
* live births per 1000 inhabitants (1988)   13,7
* population density per sq. kilometre (1987)   13
* minority groups: there has been some minor immigration from Mediterranean countries during the last decades.

(Sources: Statistical Yearbook of Norway, 1990; OECD, 1988).

The health care system

Introduction Health care in Norway is primarily the responsibility of governmental bodies. At the central government level, the Ministry of Health and Social Affairs is responsible for the organization and planning of health care. Norway's 19 counties are divided into 454 municipalities. The counties are responsible for the planning and organization of secondary health care, the municipalities for primary health care (Siem, 1986).

Health insurance Since 1967 (Siem, 1986) there is a 'National Insurance' covering social as well as health needs of all citizens. Health insurance is one of the most important items of the National Insurance. It accounted for about one third of the total expenditure on the National Insurance in 1984. The main sources of income are contributions from insurance premiums (32%) and employers contributions (46%).

In general, persons in need of medical care or other health services must pay part of the costs themselves. Drugs for chronic diseases are free, but there is co-payment for all other drugs. There is a ceiling to the total amount of user charges and for low income groups there are no co-payment obligations (Crombie et al., 1990).

Funding

Table 7.1
Total expenditure on health and public expenditure on health
(percentage of GDP)

year	total expend. % BNP	public expend. % BNP
1980	6.6	6.5
1987	7.5	7.4

Source: OECD, Health Data File, 1989

General practitioners There are two types of General Practitioners in Norway. First, there are 'municipality physicians' who are employed by the municipality and usually work in health centres. Second, there are 'private' physicians, who work in their own premises. Some of them have a contract with the municipality which provides refunding after expenditure.

The first type receives a fixed salary, the second works on an item of service basis. It is quite common for physicians to work partly in private practice and partly for the municipality.

Institutional care

Table 7.2
Number of hospital beds total and per 1000 inhabitants

years	beds total	beds per 1000
1980	29400	7.2
1981	28900	7.0
1982	27700	6.7
1983	26600	6.4
1984	25700	6.2
1985	25200	6.1
1986	25000	6.0
1987	24422	5.8

Source: Yearbook of Nordic Statistics, 1989

Community nursing

Community nursing care in Norway is provided by two types of nurses: 'hjemmesykepleier' (home nurses) who is mainly concerned with curative care, and 'helsesøster' (public health nurses), who is mainly concerned with preventive activities. Besides these two there are 'bedriftssykepleier', occupational nurses. The following description will concentrate on the 'hjemmesykepleier', the 'helsesøster', and the 'hjelpepleier' (auxiliary nurse).

History

Community nursing in Norway started in the beginning of the 19th century. Its aim was to provide care for pour people living at home. After the second world war, it was decided that health care was the responsibility of the society and should be available to all on an equal basis. Gradually a National Insurance, comparable to that in the United Kingdom, was introduced in Norway. The development of the National Insurance reached its final stage in the mid-sixties, covering all types of medical care and social services.

Until 1984, there was no unity in the organization of primary health care. Public health nurses, for example, were employed by the counties, while the municipalities covered the costs of offices and equipment. Home nursing was administered by the municipalities, but paid by the National Insurance Fund (Elstad, 1990).

With the introduction of the Municipal Health Act in 1984, the funding and organization of community nursing services has become a municipal task. According to Elstad (1990), there were several reasons for this change. Some wanted primary health care to be organized locally, as in the WHO-targets, in order to decrease the inequalities in service standards among the municipalities. Others believed that the care for the elderly would be promoted, as well as preventive health services. Still others hoped for an increasing participation of the population (ibid.).

From 1988 funding and organization of nursing homes is also a municipal task.

Organization and funding

Figure 7.1 shows the most important participants in the organization of community nursing. Most of the planning and organizational power is allocated at the local, municipality level. Municipalities are free to choose their own internal administration, they are free to determine the number of staff in primary health care, and they are free to provide extra services on top of those that are obligatory (Elstad, 1990). Communities receive a 'general block grant', covering all municipal activities. The size of this block grant is dependent on the size of the municipality, the number of elderly people, geographical circumstances and the like. Since 1986, municipalities are free to determine the proportion of this grant that should be spent on health services.

The regional level plays only a minor role where primary care is concerned, but it is not uncommon that (small) municipalities co-operate. For primary care, the only task of the regional (county) level is supervising: 'The nursing services of the county shall be under the supervision of the chief county medical officer/the chief medical officer in Oslo, who shall insure the enforcement of regulations and guidelines.' (Ministry of Health and Social Affairs, 1984).

Salaries of nurses (Table 7.3) are largely determined nationally, but there seems to be some local negotiation too, in this respect. It should be noted that there is only a very slight difference between auxiliaries and nurses.

Table 7.3
Mean gross monthly incomes of health personnel in Norwegian crowns

ward nurse	14,567
specialised nurses	14,111
nurses	12,489
health visitors/public health nurses	13,223
auxiliaries	12,127
home helps	11,307

Source: Statistical Yearbook of Norway

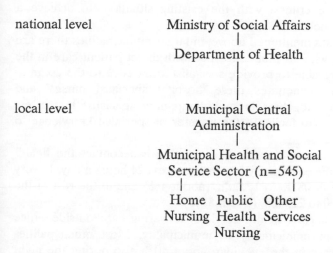

Figure 7.1 Principal participants in the planning of community nursing services

Most community nurses work from centres which house other health services as well. In most municipalities, the administration of nursing and social services (home help services) is closely linked together. Some have physio-therapists, occupational therapists, pediatrists, psychologists, physicians in addition to these services. Some of these work on a full-time basis, but usually they have a part-time contract with the community and are private practitioners in the rest of their time. In 71% of the municipalities, home help services are part of the community nursing service. However, while nursing is free of charge, home help services ask a contribution from the client (Quivey, 1989). This contribution may vary from 100 to 700 NK. a month, dependent on income (Taverne, 1990).

Large municipalities are often divided into districts. Each such district has a responsible nurse, though she frequently consults and co-operates with other nurses and/or auxiliaries. The districts vary in size and number of personnel. It is the nurse who is responsible for the care delivered to each patient in a district, even when the care is in fact delivered by an auxiliary.

The allocation of resources and the distribution of personnel in each municipality is the result of a political process at the municipality level. In Oslo, accounting for 10% of Norway's inhabitants, attempts were made to establish objective criteria, involving the age and size of the population, the number of immigrants and refugees, the number of one parent families, the closeness of the social network, the number of cases of incest and child abuse, the extent of drug abuse, the number of families moving out of or into the community, and the necessity of preventive work for the population in general, particularly the older population (Quivey, 1989). An attempt was made to combine these criteria with the existing situation, to achieve a redistribution of personnel.

In addition to the nurses mentioned above, in larger municipalities there are specialists in hospitals, who are not concerned with direct patient care in the community but who are able to provide specialist knowledge to the community nurses necessary. Sometimes these 'hospital specialist nurses' and community nurses work together in multidisciplinary specialist teams, especially created in order to facilitate the transfer of specialist knowledge to the community.

In most large municipalities (about 40%) people can contact the health service (among which the community nursing services) 24 hours a day. In very small municipalities from 08.00 to 17.00 h. (about 4%) and in the rest of the municipalities from 7.00 to 22.00 h. (about 57%).

The possibility of municipal health services delivering care outside office hours also varies from municipality to municipality. Most municipalities (about 57%) deliver care in the evenings, about 40% also during the night (some only in very urgent cases). All municipalities have a weekend-service.

Types of community nurses and manpower

Education The Norwegian registered nurse has three years basic training, including a four month's practical training. After registration as a general nurse, a 1 year's training is required to qualify for the psychiatric nurse or public health nurse or midwife's diplomas (see WHO, 1981).

One year's training, and an additional year of in-service training is needed to become a nursing auxiliary. Specialization as a psychiatric nursing auxiliary, obstetric nursing auxiliary or auxiliary for the mentally retarded, requires an extra 6 months of in-service training.

The community component in basic nursing training is currently being increased (Quivey, 1989). It was reported that students had 4 to 6 weeks of practical training in a home nursing service and 2 weeks with a public health nurse.

Manpower It was indicated before that municipalities are free to determine their own staffing ratio's for health personnel. Target ratio's therefore will vary from municipality to municipality. However, national figures exist and are presented in Table 4.

Table 7.4
Number of inhabitants per nurse in Norway in full-time equivalents in 1983
(absolute number of full-time equivalents in brackets)

	no. of inhabitants per nurse	no. of full time equivalent
nurses in non-institutional health services:	1225	(3375)
among which Nurses (specialist nurses included)	5831	(709)
home nurses	4724	(875)
head home nurse	8872	(466)
health visitors	4069	(1016)
other	13397	(309)
auxiliaries (non-institutional health services)	2804	(1474)
among which: in prophylactic service		(74)
in general practitioner service		(194)
other	3519	(1175)

Source: Statistisk Sentralbyrå, 1983

There appears to be .44 of an auxiliary for every nurse in non-institutional health services. Most of the auxiliaries work in nursing homes or homes for the elderly but these are not shown in the table.

Patient populations

Home nursing Table 7.5 shows some characteristics of the patients cared for by home nurses. It is interesting to note that, during holidays, to relieve the community nurses, it is possible that home nurses refer their patients to hospitals for some time. In these cases hospital personnel takes over part of the necessary care.

We see the largest part of the workload of home nurses being with the elderly. About 28% of the population above 80 is registered in home nursing. The population above 67 accounted for 77% of all visits in home nursing during one year (1989) (Central Bureau of Statistics of Norway, 1990). According to Hoverstad et al. (1986), this age group accounts for 83% of the total number of patients in Oslo, and for 79% of the total amount of time spent with patients.

It is interesting to note that only 2.7% of the population as a whole is registered for home-nursing. Romøren reports an even lower percentage: 2% during a year (Romøren, 1989)

Table 7.5
Patients cared for by home nurses

residence	no. of patients treated in home nursing (1988) as % of population, by age.		category
			- mentally handicapped
- home	0-16	0.1	- physically handicapped
- homes for the elderly	16-66	0.9	
	67-79	10.0	- mentally ill
- nursing homes	80-		
- hospitals (seldom)		28.8	- terminally ill
	total:	2.7	- chronically ill
			- post hospital

Source: Central Bureau of Statistics of Norway 1990; Kommunehelsetjenesten Årsstatistik, 1989

Health visitors Health visitors, who take care of the preventive activities are mainly concerned with pregnant women, mother and child care and occasionally with mentally or physically handicapped and the chronically ill. In many cases these tasks are combined with school nursing (Paulsen, 1990). About 24% of all mothers are seen during pregnancy. About 78% of all newborn children are visited within the first 4 weeks after birth (88% before the 8th week) and between 92 and 95% of all children are vaccinated in the first year (Central Bureau of Statistics of Norway, 1989). Health visitors care for elderly too, though they take up only a small percentage of their total number of clients (12.4%) (Paulsen, 1990).

Types of care

Home nurses Home nurses deliver the types of care in Table 7.6. Specialist nurses, though very common in hospitals and other institutional care settings, are very limited in numbers in community care. However, as we stated above, specialist knowledge and skills are, in some instances, transferred from institutional nurses to home nurses through specialist nurses working in hospitals.

Table 7.6
Types of care delivered by home nurses in Norway

- some health promotion (advice and providing information on for instance family planning, sex education, AIDS prevention)
- hygienic and personal care
- routine technical nursing procedures
- some more complicated technical nursing procedures
- provision of information on for instance medicine or nutrition
- psychosocial activities
- encourage help from family members etc.
- assessment of individual patient's need

The second level of expertise, auxiliaries, are mainly concerned with hygienic care, home help care, some routine nursing care, psychosocial activities, stimulation of help from family members.

According to questionnaires most of the home nurse's time is spent on home visits (60-80%), consultation hours (5-20%), administrative activities (5-25%). Preventive activities do take place, but they are difficult to estimate in terms of time, since they are combined with other care activities. Preventive home visits to elderly persons are unusual, except in some municipalities for newly retired people, to introduce them to the community nursing service. Of all visits by home nurses 88% was mainly for nursing activities, and 12% for observational activities (Central Statistical Bureau of Norway, 1990).

Head nurses are also doing home visits (5-10% of her time) and consultation hours (5-15% of her time), but most of her time (50-80%) is spent on administrative activities.

A study in Oslo (Hoverstad et al., 1986) showed the following distribution of nursing activities:

Table 7.7
Percentage of working time of home nurses spent on selected activities

distribution of indirect care (51% of total time):		distribution of direct care (49% of total time):	
office work	25%	admission visits	2%
meetings	25%	physical care (hygienic)	42%
in-service education	4%	nutrition	8%
travel	30%	medicine	8%
miscellaneous	14%	procedures (technical)	15%
other	2%	general observ.	6%
		mental care	15%
	100%	assistance	2%
		other	2%
			100%

Source: Hoverstad et al, 1986

It appears from the table that equal parts of the total working time are spent on direct and indirect care and that, in direct care, most time is spent on physical care, technical procedures and mental care.

Auxiliaries Auxiliaries also spend most of their time (55-80%) on home visits. They very seldom do consultation hours, and spend very little of their time on administrative activities.

Health visitors Health visitors are primarily concerned with activities listed in Table 7.8.

Table 7.8
Activities of health visitors

- health promotion
- assessment of groups at risk
- providing information on for instance medicine or nutrition
- psychosocial activities
- stimulate help from family members
- assessment of individual patient's need

Health visitors sometimes have tasks in school nursing and health centres. The percentages of the total health centre time spent on some activities are shown in Table 7.9.

Table 7.9
Percentage of total health center time spent on selected activities by health visitors (N=68)

consultations with mothers and newborns	37%
administrative	37%
home visits	11%
telephone conversations with clients	7%
other	8%
total	100

Source: Paulsen, 1990

Only 11% percent of the total health center time is spent on home visits. Home visits only take place for the very young children.

General There is no statutory maximum to the amount of care delivered by either health visitors or home nurses. The maximum amount of care is dependent on the available resources and the patient's need.

Stages in nursing

Home nursing According to the community health statistics (Central Statistical Bureau of Norway, 1990) 70% of the first contacts is initiated by the patient him/herself, his family or general practitioner. About 30% is referred by hospital nursing homes or other institutes. Although a standardised referral form is used, no exact data on this topic are available. No referrals are made by home help organizations, since they are part of the community nursing service in most municipalities.

Assessment visits are exclusively done by home nurses or head nurses. Assessment for nursing care and home help care is combined in those municipalities where home help and nursing services take part in the same organization. Assessment is made using forms for activities of daily living, like dressing, washing, cooking, as well as forms for assessment of the psychological/social status of the patient, including items like 'able to read', 'being forgetful', 'need for social contact', 'receiving help from others', etc. In these forms there is an opportunity to state the time needed from health or social services to relieve the need for help. In addition, there is the option to evaluate the patient's needs on this form.

The head nurse or home nurse decides whether a first level home nurse or an auxiliary is going to deliver the care and nurses are responsible for their own actions.

Health visiting According to Paulsen (1990) about 70% of all consultations is initiated by the nurse herself and about 30% by the patient herself. In most cases the health visitor works solo, without physicians present at consultation hours. Each child is subject to a vaccination and screening program.

Relations with general practitioners, home help services and hospitals
Community nursing services, home help services and GP services are part of the same organization in most municipalities. Consequently there is frequent co-operation between these services. In addition, co-operation takes place with hospitals, psychiatric services and nursing homes. In Nord Odal, a village with 5500 inhabitants, (Taverne, 1990) nurses met weekly with other health personnel (physicians, physiotherapist, occupational therapists and home helps). In this community home care is co-ordinated by a specially appointed 'head of home care' (ibid.). It must be noted, however, that the municipality of Nord Odal is not representative for Norway as such, since it takes part in a series of experiments in community care in Norway (Bølstad and Melbye, 1990).

General practitioners and community nurses have frequent face to face contact and meetings to discuss individual patients/clients and to discuss service referrals. The number of GPs that an individual nurse has to deal with varies from municipality to municipality. The nurse may have to deal with all GPs in the community, but it is also possible that she only has to deal with some of them. Usually contact with the municipality's doctor takes place more often than with a 'private doctor' (see page 120).

Probably contacts with home help services are even more frequent, since in 71% of the communities, these services are administered by the community nursing services. As indicated before, the home nurse who carries out the assessment visit may also determine that the patient needs home help care. No problems were reported concerning the division of tasks between home helps and nursing personnel.

Though nursing homes usually have so-called liaison nurses, they are not very common in hospitals. Some acute somatic hospitals, however, are very slowly introducing this or discussing it.

Problems

Underperformance There were several activities that were regarded as underperformed:
- psychosocial activities;
- encouragement of help from family members, neighbours etc., mainly

with elderly;
- home help care for mothers and new babies and elderly;
- preventive activities for the elderly.

Personnel shortages There appears to be a shortage of nursing personnel of 10%, mainly in nursing homes. This is partly due to the fact that many nurses (about 50%) work only part time (Bunch, 1988). Bunch forecasts an overall shortage of nurses of 49% in the year 2006. Quivey (1989) suspects the shortage of home care nurses is due to the fact that nursing students spend a rather limited time in community nursing during their studies. Others think there is just not enough money to create the necessary services. As one of our contacts put it: 'First they (the government) give us (the local authorities) full responsibility, and subsequently they give us not enough money to do it'. On the other hand, Quivey (ibid.) states that 'Over the last 10 years, adequate budget for home care services has not been a major problem. There is political agreement to give these services top priority. When the services still are not satisfactory in some areas of the country it is due to difficulties in recruitment'.

Waiting lists for community nursing care are not really a problem. A research project in Oslo revealed waiting times varying from 0 to 10 days. However, according to one of the consulted experts, the non-existence of a problem in this respect is mainly due to the strict selectivity regarding acceptance on the waiting list. In other words: one has to be quite needy before being allowed on to a waiting list.

Specialist versus generalist No problems were reported on the division of tasks between public health nurses and home nurses.

Levels of expertise and home helps No problems were reported on the division of tasks between nurses and auxiliaries.

Home help and community nursing take often part in the same organization. No problems were reported on the division of tasks between nurses and home helps.

Community nursing and general practitioner Community nursing and general practitioner services are both part of the same organization. No problems were reported on the division of tasks.

Hospital and community nursing Though nursing homes often employ liaison nurses, this is not the case in most hospitals. In some hospitals this issue is discussed.

Funding According to some experts too few funds are allocated to community nursing services to be able to maintain enough personnel. However, Quivey (1989) states that money has not been a problem in the last ten years.

Other problems Comparing the status of community nursing in Norway with the Vienna Declaration on Nursing, Quivey (1989) discerns 3 potentially problematic areas. She wants to give priority to:
- increasing the community component in basic nursing education;
- increasing nursing research in community nursing, particularly in the clinical area;
- increasing community participation to make sure we develop the kind of services the Norwegian people wants.

References

Bölstad, J., B. Melbye (1990), *Sosialdepartementets omsorgsserie 1/90, Omsorgstjenester i utvikling; Program og prosjekter* [Health and socialservices in development programs and projects], Sosialdepartementet, Oslo.

Bunch, E.H. (1988), *Manpower Study; are they helpful and what can they tell us?* Paper presented at WENR, June 26-29.

Central Bureau of Statistics of Norway (1990), *Rapporter 90/18, Kommunehelsetjenesten for 1989* [Community health care for 1989], Oslo-Kongsvinger.

Elstad, J.I. (1990), 'Health services and decentralized government: the case of primary health services in Norway', *International Journal of Health Services*, 20, 4, pp. 545-559.

Hoverstad, L., A. Johansen, M. Quivey (1986), *Analyse av virksomhet i hjemmesykepleien* [Analysis of the functioning of home nursing], Helserad, rapport no 3, Oslo.

Ministry of Health and Social Affairs (1983), *Regulations concerning statutory nursing in the municipal health service*, Oslo.

Paulsen, B. (1990). *Snakk med de på helsestationen; en analyse av bruk av helsesøstertjenesten* [Talking to people in health centers; an analysis of the use of the helsesøster], Oslo: Norsk institutt for sykehusforskning, NIS-RAPPRT 3.

Quivey, M. (1989), *Community nursing in Norway*, In: A. Kerkstra, R. Verheij, Community nursing; proceedings of the international conference on community nursing 16-17 March 1989, NIVEL, Utrecht.

Romoren, T.I. (1989), *Kommunehelsetjenestens fem første år* [The first five years of community health care], Sosialdepartementet Helseavdelingen, Rapport no. 12, Oslo.

Siem, H. (1986), *Choices for Health; an introduction to the health services in Norway*, Oslo: Universitetsforlaget.

Statistisk Sentralbyrå (1990), *Statistical yearbook 1990*, Oslo-Kongsvinger.

Statistisk Semtralbyrå (1984), *Statistics on health personnel 1983*, Oslo-Kongsvinger.

Taverne, M (1990), Thuiszorg werkt in Noorwegen [Home care works in Norway], *Fysiovisie*, mei.

References

8 Community nursing in England

The setting [1] [2]

Population [3]
* total population Great Britain & N. Ireland (1987) 56,9 million
* % over 65 (1987)   15,3
* % over 65 (2000, projected)   14,5
* % over 65 (2010, projected)   14,6
* % over 65 (2020, projected)   16,3
* % under 15 (1987)   18,9
* life expectancy at birth (1985-87) (England & Wales) 71,9 (men)
                                                       77,6 (women)
* live births per 1000 inhabitants (1988)   13,8
* population density per sq. kilometre (1987)   233
* population groups: some cultural minorities from Mediterranean countries and former British colonies.

Health care system

Introduction The United Kingdom is a constitutional monarchy consisting of four countries; England, Wales, Scotland and Northern Ireland. The four countries enjoy a considerable degree of autonomy in areas such as education, health, housing and social policy.

At the local level there are differences in structure of the health services between England and the three other countries. This description concentrates on England.

A few years ago the former Department of Health and Social Services (DHSS) was split up into a Department of Health and a Department of Social Services.

Today, at the national level, the Department of Health is in charge of the formulation of policies in relation to health, the assessments of needs, the allocation of resources and the definition of priorities. The Department of Health allocates funds and is accountable for them to Parliament.

At the regional level, in England 14 Regional Health Authorities (RHAs) have three main tasks:
- directing management of the district i.e. resource allocation, assessing of needs and monitor the functioning of services;
- building hospitals;
- defining and implementing ten-year strategic plans, which broadly follow Department of Health policies.

At the local level, 192 District Health Authorities (DHAs) manage the local health services and assess the local needs. They also define and implement operational plans for their area (see also figure 8.1)

About 90 Family Health Services Authorities (FHSAs) also operate at the local level. They administer the national contracts with GPs, GDPs (dentists), pharmacists and opticians. The FHSAs are appointed by the Secretary of State and consist of 30 members of whom 15 come from the professions concerned, the other 15 members are laymen.

From April 1991 the Regional Health Authorities will assume responsibility for allocating cash-limited resources for GP practice staff to FHSAs as well as to the district health authorities (North West Thames Regional Health Authority, 1991).

Arrangements are similar in Wales, but in Scotland and Northern Ireland, Health Boards have the same function as DHAs and FHSAs.

Health insurance All citizens of the UK have been covered by a National Health Service (NHS) since 1948. The NHS provides free primary and hospital care, although there are some patient charges for prescribed drugs, dental care and some appliances. There is a small private sector, providing mainly acute hospital service involving elective surgery, which is supplementary to the NHS.

Financing The English NHS is divided into 3 sectors: (1) the hospital and community health services (HCHS), (2) the family practitioner services (FPS) and (3) the local authority (government) social services (LASS).

The HCHS budget is cash limited and divided amongst the RHAs by a formula (Resource Allocation Working Party, RAWP) based on population weighted by standardized mortality ratios. Each RHA has discretion as to how it distributes resources amongst their DHAs.

The FPS budget finances ambulatory medical care. This budget is 'open-ended' and demand determined, i.e., expenditure is determined by the practices of GPs and other practitioners contracted to the FPS to provide services for patients.

LASSs are funded from local taxes and central government grants. Local government is controlled extensively by central government. The LASS budget is cash limited and there is an element of equalization of financial capacity by central government in that their grants for LASS, the rate support grant, has a 'needs' element in it.

Table 8.1
Total and public expenditure on health care in Great Britain
(percent of GDP)

year	total expend. % GDP	public expend. % GDP	expend. in £ per head
1980	5.78	5.18	237
1981	6.05	5.40	273
1982	5.94	5.22	292
1983	6.16	5.40	330
1984	6.11	5.33	349
1985	5.99	5.20	373
1986	6.02	5.22	400
1987	6.05	5.23	435

Source: Program ECO-SANTE by BASYS/CREDES

General practitioners [4] The whole population has direct access to general medical and dental practitioners (GPs and GDPs), pharmacists and opticians. GPs (but not GDPs) maintain a list of patients for whom they are responsible; a patient may choose any practitioner subject to their being willing to take the patient on their list. GPs act as gatekeeper to specialist services, regulating access to non-emergency hospital services. They work mainly in group-practices (70%) or partnerships (18%), as well as in multidisciplinary health centres (25%). Only 12% work in solo practices. GPs, GDPs [5] and pharmacists are not directly employed by the NHS, but are independent practitioners under contract with the NHS (they are called 'independent contractors').

GP remuneration is a mix of fees and practice allowances; most of these fees are, however, based on capitation rather than fee-for-service. A GP receives standard capitation fees based on the number of patients on his list and receives fees for new patients. Besides that a GP can receive extra payments for childhood immunisation, cervical screening, minor surgery and some other items.

137

There are .56 general practitioners per 1000 inhabitants (1986 National Yearbook). 15% of all patient contacts involve home visits.

Institutional care   Hospital services are also provided as part of the NHS. These services are free of charge. According to the type and severity of the illness the services may be provided on an inpatient, outpatient or day-patient basis.

In contrast to general practitioners, specialist are salaried and hospital based. There is a relatively small number of beds in private hospitals. Patients should be referred by a GP to receive hospital care.

Mean length of stay in somatic hospitals in days (1980) (OECD, 1987): 13.3.

Table 8.2
Inpatient medical care beds and personnel per bed

years total	beds per 1000	beds per bed	personnel
1980	458000	8.1	1.40
1981	455000	8.1	1.50
1982	453000	8.0	1.53
1983	446400	7.9	1.58
1984	430815	7.6	1.64
1985	421195	7.4	1.71
1986	409962	7.2	1.76
1987	388711	6.8	1.86

Source: Program ECO-SANTE by BASYS/CREDES

Community nursing

Community nursing in England is mainly provided by district nurses and health visitors. In the following description community psychiatric nurses were included, because they are a growing group of nurses in the community. There are three levels of expertise: registered nurses, enrolled nurses and auxiliaries.

Before discussing the tasks and other characteristics of these nurses, first the history, organization and financing of community nursing in England will be described.

District nursing as well as health visiting started in the second half of the 19th century following the cholera epidemic in the area of Manchester. The purpose was to offer home care to all sick people, not just the rich. In 1948 district nursing as well as health visiting became part of the National Health Service.

Initially concerned with promoting health and hygiene for the population in general, health visiting began to focus more and more on child health during the first half of the 20th century, when infant mortality was very high. Today a re-emergence of the public health movement is taking place, in which health visiting should focus more on the population in general.

Organization and financing

Department of Health
|
14 Regional Health Authorities
|
192 District Health
Authorities'
Community Units
|
Localities / Neighbourhoods / Sectors
|
Health Centre

Figure 8.1 Planning hierarchy of community health services in England

District nurses, as well as health visitors are paid a salary by the District Health Authorities (DHAs). Gross incomes vary roughly between £ 7,000 and £ 20,000 yearly.

Each DHA has a community unit - a sort of department of community care - which is divided into several localities, neighbourhoods or sectors. Localities and neighbourhoods are created according to a functional criterion (for instance areas of deprivation, or areas with mainly local authority housing), sectors according to a more rigid geographical criterion by simply dividing, an area, for example, into a number of equal parts.

For each locality, neighbourhood or sector there is a manager who is responsible for staff deployment in that area, in which there may be several health centres.

Most district nurses work from health centres, though this does not necessarily mean that nurses work from health centres on a daily basis. According to

Dunnel and Dobbs (1982) 61% of all district nurses and 6% of all health visitors regard their home as their work base, but according information in the questionnaire there has been a change towards health centres in the last decade regarding district nurses. Most community psychiatric nurses work from hospitals (49.2%)(White, 1990).

Several health services may be provided from health centres, including district nursing, health visiting, general practice, chiropodist, and school nursing. Large differences exist between health centres in this respect.

The population that is served by a health centre as well as the number of personnel varies dependent on area. There are no national regulations in this respect, though some target ratio's have been formulated.

It should be remembered that the NHS is in the midst of a major organizational reform, creating an internal market for health care providers. 'Nurses in the community setting will operate within a system of a Government funded, internal market, offering contracted work to budget holding health authorities and family doctors or to private health care facilities' (Butterworth, 1990). This implies that in the future community nurses (district nurses as well as health visitors) may be employed by one of several different organizations.

A choice for one of these organizations - NHS trusts, Family Health Services Authority, budget holding GPs, district health authorities (see North West Th. Regional Health Authority, 1990) - will be made by the local authorities (see appendix 4). Consequently the outcome will vary locally.

Since the outcome of this reorganization is still unclear, this description will be limited to the situation in February 1991.

Types of community nurses and manpower

General In the UK there are several types of nurses working in the community. The most important ones are:
- district nurses;
- health visitors;
- community psychiatric nurses;
- school nurses;
- GP practice nurses.

There are three levels of expertise: registered nurses and enrolled nurses and auxiliaries (see below).

This description will focus on district nurses, health visitors and community psychiatric nurses.

In addition to the nurses mentioned above, there are some district nurses who have specialized in specific types of care, such as stoma or diabetic nurses. Most of these nurses have a consultative role towards the other personnel, but are also concerned with direct patient care. Some of these specialist nurses work in both hospital and community units.

There are also specialist health visitors for example for children with special learning needs. These health visitors work at the district health authority level and are usually concerned with direct patient care and may visit jointly with family health visitors.

Secondly there are nurse managers with specialist knowledge who are not concerned with direct patient care but advise and support health visitors on all matters relating to child protection.

Basic education   In Britain there are three basic types of nursing education: registered nurses, enrolled nurses, and auxiliaries. The first with three years of education, the second with two, and the third with no need for formal qualifications. Most nursing schools are attached to a major hospital, though there are 8 universities (in 1985-6, Hoad, 1987) offering nursing qualification: registration as a nurse as well as an academic degree.

Further education   There are many possibilities for further education at various institutes and with a varying duration. Additional qualifications can be for instance in community psychiatry, health visiting, district nursing, obstetrics, orthopaedics, family planning, mental handicapped, occupational health, school health.

In their 1980 study Dunnell and Dobbs (1982) found the most common post registration qualifications to be the family planning certificate, the midwifery qualification and the district nursing certificate, even where they were not directly related to the nurse's current job. 61% of all district nurses was in the possession of a district nursing certificate, 25% had a midwifery qualification, 99% of all health visitors had a health visitors certificate (not very surprising, since it is a statutory requirement to have a HV certificate before one can practice health visiting). In 1990 34.6% of the CPN workforce in England had completed a one-year psychiatric nursing course (White, 1990).

A post-registration health visiting certificate can be obtained by following a 51-week course at a college of higher education, at a university or a polytechnic. District nurse post-registration courses can be followed at these same institutes and takes 9 months (2/3 practice and 1/3 theory).

For enrolled nurses there is a 4-6 month course in district nursing.

Trends in education   It should be remembered that education in nursing in the UK is currently being reformed. In the new educational program, which is called project 2000, one of the most important developments is that the second level (enrolled) nurse is being phased out. This type of education will simply cease to exist. There is going to be only one 3 year educational scheme with specializations in the last 18 months.

It is, however, realised that there is a need for second level personnel and

141

therefore the term 'support worker' has been invented. Though this is not at all certain yet, their training will probably take 2 years. Probably there will also be different grades in this training.

Another important development is increasing emphasis on nursing in the community in the new educational program. Nurses will be trained better to deal with 'real people' in stead of 'patients' and will therefore go out more into the community during their training.

Manpower The total numbers of nurses in England from 1985 to 1989 are shown in tabel 8.3. The second level of expertise appears to be mainly working as a district nurse. Among district nurses there appears to be about 0.5 enrolled nurse for every registered nurse. There are hardly any enrolled health visitors.

Table 8.3
Number of nurses in England in 1985, 1986, 1987, 1988 and 1989
in full-time equivalents

	1985	1986	1987	1988	1989
health visiting:					
health visitors	10.240	10.393	10.333	10.313	--
other registered*	871	460	641	689	--
other enrolled*	100	93	91	102	--
student health visitors	866	832	785	786	--
other nursing staff	204	224	260	235	--
district nursing:					
district nurses	8.998	9.119	8.691	8.648	--
district nursing tutorial	50	43	43	42	--
other registered*	1.876	1.315	1.732	1.763	--
other enrolled*	4.216	4.296	4.232	4.221	--
student district nurses	704	680	650	608	--
other nursing staff	2.998	3.203	3.300	3.265	--
school nursing service:					
registered nurses	2.493	2.485	2.473	2.415	--
enrolled nurses	189	182	162	142	--
community psychiatric nursing (part-time CPNs excluded)	--	--	--	--	3.730

* = nurses without district nursing resp. health visiting certificate.

Sources: Department of Health, 1990; White, 1990

142

In 1972, the DHSS stated a general target ratio for district nurses of 1:4000 and 1:2,500 in area's with a large elderly population or extensive attachments (Baker et al., 1987). The targets for health visitors were 1:4,300 and 1:3,000 in area's with extensive attachments and/or high immigrant population (ibid.).

For community psychiatric nurses, most commonly, the target ratio's were between 1:10.000 to 1:12.000 (White, 1990). If we add the various types of district nurses, health visitors and school nurses, listed in tabel 8.3, we come to the nurse-population ratios in tabel 8.4.

Tabel 8.4
Number of inhabitants per nurse, for health visitors, district nurses and registered school nurses and community psychiatric nurses in England in 1988 (full-time equivalents)

health visitors	4.609
district nurses	5.497
registered school nurses	19.683
community psychiatric nurses	12.700 (in 1990)

Source: Department of Health, 1990; White, 1990; own computations

It appears from tabel 8.4 that these targets have not been reached. It must be noted, however, that auxiliaries are not included in these figures.

Unfortunately, national figures on auxiliary manpower were not available. Some indication in this respect, however, may be given by a study in the district nursing service of Wycombe in 1986 (Finlay et al., 1986). In this district there was .5 auxiliary for every district nurse.

Patient populations

District nurses It can be seen from table 8.5 that district nurses care for people in their own homes, but also in old people's homes without registered nursing staff. These old people's homes provide only minimal care for their residents, consisting mainly of ADL care and the provision of meals. For nursing care, people have to turn to district nurses. We were informed that in the area of Manchester old people's homes are shooting up like mushrooms and that there is no formal qualification needed to establish one. Consequently there are good ones and bad ones.

Most patients, or clients, as some district nurses prefer to call them, are over 65 years of age. Children make up only a small part of the patient population, since the healthy children are cared for by health visitors (see below) and district nurses only care for sick children.

Table 8.5
Patients cared for by district nurses

residence	persons treated (first treatment) by age, 1987/88 (n=3,459,600)		category
- home	< 5	3.8	- mentally
- home for the	5-16	5.4	handicapped
elderly	17-64	43.5	- physically
	> 65	47.3	handicapped
	total	100%	- mentally ill
			- terminally ill*
	Source: Department		- chronically ill
	of Health, 1990		- post-hospital

*) For the terminally ill, there is a separate organization, a MacMillan fund, which provides extra nursing, in addition to the normal provision.

Per 1000 of the population in England, 73 persons were cared for by district nursing services (Department of Health, 1990).

According to Dunnell and Dobbs (1982), there is very little difference between registered and enrolled nurses in respect of the amount of time spent with specific age groups and patient categories. Auxiliaries, however, are more concerned with the physical problems than enrolled nurses or registered nurses, but spend as much time on elderly patients.

Health visitors Health visitors take care of the healthy population. Most of their workload consists of children (table 8.6) and their mothers, though they claim to provide care from the cradle to the grave. Care for the elderly population usually takes place in the form of courses on how to live a healthy life and how to cope with the problems of becoming older. In addition, there are some "well-elderly" screening programmes and follow-up following discharge from hospital or following bereavement.

A decreasing percentage of the population above 65 is visited by health visitors (7.4% in 1978 and 5.3% in 1987/88) (Department of Health, 1990). According to Dunnell and Dobbs (1982) only 9% of the health visitor's time was spent with elderly patients.

Table 8.6
Persons cared for by health visitors

residence	persons visited at home (first visits) by age, 1987/88 (n=4.093.000)		category
- home	births	18%	- pregnant women
	1-4	38%	- mothers and new
	5-6	5%	babies
	17-64	29%	- well elderly clients
	> 65	10%	
	total	100%	

Source: Department of Health, 1990

In 1987/88 8.6% of the total population were visited by health visitors (Department of Health 1990). In addition to home visits, 94% of all births were seen in child health clinics in the year they were born (Department of Health, 1990).

Community psychiatric nursing The workload of CPNs mostly comprises mentally ill adults. In England 47.9 % of the clients had previous psychiatric admission, 42.6% concerned chronically ill persons and 26% cases of schizophrenia (White, 1990).

A large proportion of CPNs reported specializing in a particular client group. In England this was 44.4% (White, 1990). Most of these specialize in care for the elderly (about 60%, ibid). Some 10% specialized in drugs/alcohol and about 17% in rehabilitation/resettlement.

Types of care

District nursing District nurses take care of the entire sick population in a specific area (see table 8.7). In some cases, however, there are specialist nurses in for instance stoma care or diabetes (see above)

Table 8.7
Types of care delivered by registered district nurses

-     health promotion (advice)
-     assessment of groups at risk in the community
-     hygienic and personal care
-     routine technical nursing procedures
-     more complicated technical nursing procedures
-     provision of information on for instance medicine or nutrition
-     **some** psychosocial activities
-     encourage help from family members etc.

There are no government or other regulations stating the maximum amount of care a patient is entitled to receive.

The second level of expertise, enrolled nurses, are primarily concerned with hygienic and other personal care, routine technical nursing, and stimulation of help from others.

Auxiliaries are primarily concerned with hygienic and other personal care.

It was impossible to give exact recent data on the percentage of time spent on selected activities. It was estimated that registered and enrolled nurses spend about 70% of their time on home visits, whereas auxiliaries spend about 90% of their time on home visits (figures include time spent on travelling). Registered nurses spend about 25% of their time on paperwork, enrolled nurses about 10% and auxiliaries about 5%. Preventive activities are usually carried out by registered nurses.

Similar results appeared in a study of the district nursing service of the Wycombe Health Authority (Findlay et al., 1986). Registered and enrolled nurses spent 51% of their time on home visits; 19% on travelling; 5% on treatment sessions; 24% non-patient contact time. In this study, however it appeared that enrolled nurses spent as much time as the registered nurse on administrative activities.

Health visiting Health visitors take care of the whole healthy population. However, they work mainly with children and their families.

Table 8.8
Types of care delivered by health visitors

-   health promotion
-   assessment of groups at risk
-   providing information about for instance medicine, nutrition
-   psychosocial activities (discussing psychosocial problems, advising)
-   encourage help from family members
-   immunisations

Health visitors spend all of their time on preventive activities. With the exception of immunization, health visitors rarely perform practical nursing tasks.

It is impossible to give figures on the percentage of time spent on home visits, administration, consultation hours or the time spent in clinics. It has to be noted that consultation hours are usually not set and that patients usually make contact by telephone when they need the help of a health visitor.

Child health clinic sessions are held by a health visitor alone in 38% of the sessions. In the rest of the cases a physician is present too.

Community psychiatric nursing Community psychiatric nurses are nurses who specialize in the mentally ill. They are concerned with
-   health promotion
-   assessment of groups at risk in the community
-   hygienic and other personal care
-   routine technical nursing procedures
-   providing information on medicine, nutrition
-   psychosocial activities
-   encouragement of help from family members
-   **some** home help type care

Community psychiatric nurses are increasingly offering psychotherapeutic skills. In 1990 15.3% (White, 1990) of the community psychiatric nurses in England reported to specialize with a specific therapeutic approach like family therapy (28%), behaviour therapy (19.5%) and counselling (12.8%) (ibid).

Stages in nursing

District nursing There are several ways in which contact with a patient is initiated (table 8.9).

Table 8.9
Percentage of patients with whom the first contact is initiated by (estimates):

patient him/herself or family	5%
general practitioner	40%
home help services	5%
hospital or nursing home for elderly	40%
other professional care providers	10%

Source: questionnaire

Please note the high proportion of patients whose contact with district nurses is initiated by hospitals or nursing homes. It is impossible to state anything about the ratio between hospitals and nursing homes. In the Wycombe study (Findley et al., 1986) 70% of all patients were referred by their GP, whilst only 17.5% by hospitals. The conclusion may be that these figures probably have a large variation dependent on area.

Assessment visits are done by registered nurses. Usually no check lists are used doing this. Assessment is not in this way standardized although some experiments have been carried out in this respect (see Baker et al., 1987). The decision who is going to give the care is also made by the registered nurse. She can also decide that home help is needed and mediate between patient and home help service. The district nurse is always responsible for the actions she delegates to enrolled nurses and auxiliaries.

Informal evaluation usually takes place each new visit. Formal evaluation or reassessment will vary dependent on the case and is carried out by registered nurses only.

Health visiting Child delivery in the UK usually takes place in (maternity) hospitals. Home deliveries are rare. This is the reason why most of the health visitor's patients were referred by maternity hospitals (table 8.10).

Table 8.10
Estimate of the percentage of the total number of patients with whom the first contact is initiated by:

patient him/herself or family	30-35%
general practitioner	10-15%
(maternity) hospital	50-60%

Source: questionnaire

In contrast to district nurses, health visitors do follow guidelines for assessment of a child's health and check whether the child is developing normally.

Community psychiatric nursing Most of the community psychiatric nurse's workload is referred to them by psychiatrists (table 8.11). Between 1985 and 1990, however, the general practitioner became more important in this respect. (23.3% and 35.8% respectively).

No checklists are used to assess the patient's health.

Table 8.11
Distribution of sources of client referral to community psychiatric nurses
(1990)

psychiatrist	42.7
general practitioner	35.8
district nurse / health visitor	3.9
hospital staff	5.5
social services	3.6
relatives / self	4.4
other	4.1

Source: White, 1990

Relations with general practitioners, home help services and hospitals

General Relations to other health providers in England are a matter of primary concern since the UK is in the midst of a major reorganization of the total primary care system (see appendix 4).

District nurses Most district nurses work GP attached. This means that their patient population is the same as that of one or more specific GPs. This system is possible since, due to the reimbursement according to the number of patients in their practice, GPs in the UK keep a list of their patients, contrary to for example Germany, France and Belgium. The average district nurse has to deal with 2 to 3 general practices. It is hard to state anything in general about the frequency of contact between GPs and nurses. But considering the fact that a prescription from a GP is needed for medical interventions, it can be assumed that there is frequent contact between GPs and nurses. In their 1982 study, Dunnell and Dobbs found 60% of all district nurses to have contact with a GP more than 5 times a week.

Cumberlege et al (1986) demonstrated that working GP attached has the disadvantage that the patients of a GP do not live in a geographically defined area, causing ineffective use of community nursing services because a relatively large amount of travelling time is involved.

It has to be noted that a debate is in progress about nurses prescribing and that several experiments have been carried out in this respect (see Baker et al., 1987, pp. 168-69; Butterworth, 1990, Smith, 1991, Rawlings, 1991) and that it is probable that nurses will be allowed limited prescription authority in the near future. A bill based on the Report of the Advisory Group on Nurse Prescribing (Department of Health, 1989) is currently being discussed in Parliament. The Report makes quite specified proposals on nurse prescribing.

Furthermore, it has to be noted that changes are occurring in the organization of health care. One new development is GP contracting. In this scheme a GP receives a certain budget from the NHS, allowing him/her to buy services from other health providers, among which district nurses. This means that GPs will increasingly be the centre of health care. At the moment it is not certain how district nursing will fit into the new order. It is anticipated that roles that were previously restricted to district nurses will be increasingly taken over by practice nurses employed by GPs. They are involved in treatments, screening and advice giving to patients in doctor's surgeries and increasingly in screening the elderly (by law every >75 has to be visited by a GP).

Home help services in England are not (yet?) considered to be a part of the health care system at the local level, and consequently operate independently from the NHS. These services are locally organized and their funding varies locally. In general they charge individual patients dependent on their income. Usually a district nurse only has to deal with one home help service. There is no regular contact between nurses and home help services. Here too, however, there is a tendency to take over roles previously restricted to district nurses: giving basic care, assisting particularly the elderly with help bathing, dressing, etc.

The previously mentioned change in the organization of community care, however, will also have effects on the relations between social services on the one hand and health services on the other. District health authorities, family health services associations and local authority social services departments will probably co-operate more in the future. In this view, it is interesting to note that at the national level the Department of Health and Social Services has recently been split into a Department of Health and a Department of Social Services.

It could be seen from table 8.9 that a relatively large proportion of contacts between district nurses and patients is established by hospitals, implying that contacts with hospitals are frequent. Many hospitals employ so-called liaison nurses, who take care of the continuity of care between primary and secondary care. According to expert information, there has been an increasing interest in 'hospital at home' schemes following the French model of H.à.D.

('hospitalisation à domicile', see France) which allow earlier discharge from hospital.

Health visiting Like district nurses, health visitors usually work GP attached (Baker et al., 1987). Their patient population is the same as that of a specific GP. Dunnell and Dobbs (1982) reported 89% of all health visitors to have contact with a GP at least weekly. One health visitor usually has to deal with 1-3 practices. In 62% of the child health clinic sessions the health visitor co-operates with a physician.

Health visitors may also work geographically attached. In this case contact with GPs may be less frequent and health visitors may have to deal with 20 practices.

The future of relations with GPs is uncertain. As noted earlier, GPs are increasingly becoming the centre of ambulatory care and consequently, practice nurses are increasingly taking over the roles previously exclusively restricted to health visitors. This trend is encouraged by the government, for example in demanding that every GP make an assessment visit to every patient above 75 years of age, a potential client group for preventive services. Immunizations are also increasingly being performed by general practitioners or their nurses.

Health visitors consult home help services infrequently, only when clients need referral to this service or when extra help is required. Usually health visitors have to deal with only one local social services department.

Liaison health visitors are employed by the district health authority. They take on liaison work with casualty departments in hospitals and out-patient clinics, as well as ordinary health visitor duties.

Community psychiatric nursing There is co-operation on a regular basis between community psychiatric nurses and social worker, occupational therapists, psychologists and voluntary agencies. No data were available on the frequency of contact between these services. Table 8.12, however, shows that most community psychiatric nurses have an operational base in which other care providers are housed as well, implying a high probability of contact between them.

Table 8.12
Operational base of community psychiatric nurses in England

psychiatric hospital	18.4
psychiatric unit at general hospital	15.7
general practitioner practice	21.3
day hospital	9.1
community mental health centre	20.8
other	14.7

Source: White, 1990

Problems

Underperformance First of all, it appears that nurses are not allowed to perform some more complex tasks. On the other hand, there are no legal objections to family members, neighbours or anyone who has followed a course in these matters in hospital doing these things.

Secondly, there appears to be a need for more encouragement of help from family members, neighbours and friends for mentally handicapped and the mentally ill.

Thirdly, there seems to be a need for more home help care, hygienic care, and preventive care for the elderly, a need that was already recognized by Dunnell and Dobbs (1982).

Fourthly, there seems to be a need for more home help care for the mentally handicapped (see also Dunnell and Dobbs, 1982).

Health visitors work under increasing pressure and therefore crisis work like child protection has to take priority over the preventive and developmental work with families and the community as a whole.

Personnel shortages There is no shortage of district nurses, provided that they are more effectively utilized by delegating less esoteric care to lower staff. The number of students entering district nurse courses, however, showed a decrease of 6.5% between 1985/86 and 1989/90 (English National Board for Nursing, Midwifery and Health Visiting, 1991).

A reduction of the number of health visitors is taking place while caseloads are being frozen. The decrease is visible in statistics provided by the English National Board for Nursing, Midwifery and Health Visiting (1991), which indicate a 3% decrease in the number of students entering health visiting courses between 1985/86 and 1989/90.

Specialist versus generalist According to Kerkstra (1991) preventive care for elderly suffers from the division of tasks between health visitors and district

152

nurses. According to some the artificial division between healthy and ill elderly is not very efficient and they plead for district nurses to take care of the healthy elderly too (Ross, 1985; 1987; Slater, 1987).

Furthermore, in times of limited financial resources, preventive care is easily considered to be a luxury and becomes subject to government savings (Fatchett, 1990). Finally, district nurses and health visitors usually work in seperate teams, so that they know little of each other's activities (Cumberlege, e.a., 1986).

Levels of expertise and home helps It is interesting to note that in the new educational scheme (see 'Trends in education') the second level of expertise (enrolled nurses) is being phased out and that from now on nursing schools will only produce fully qualified nurses (registered nurses). In their 1986 report, Cumberlege et al. pointed out that enrolled nurses 'have a clear and important role in community nursing. Their training enables them to carry out a wide range of cuties which can be delegated to them after proper assessment by the fully qualified community nurse.'

Phasing out of enrolled education is being carried out to elevate the status of the nursing profession and to remove a level of nurse who is being achieved by grading new staff at a lower level providing a clinical hierarchy. A new grade ('support worker') will be introduced that will presumably equate somewhere between an auxiliary and a state enrolled nurse.

There is some discussion about whether 'medical baths' should be taken care of by nurses or home helps. There is a tendency to assign home helps to the delivery of hygienic care.

Community nursing and general practitioner Most district nurses and health visitors work GP-attached. The advantage seems to be that there are better opportunities for co-operation. The disadvantage is that longer travelling is involved because the patients of GPs do not live geographically concentrated.

Recent government publications indicate a wish to make the GP the pivot in health care (for instance HMSO, 1987).

The division of tasks between health visitors and GPs and/or practice nurses is problematic, since many preventive tasks are taken over by GPs or their practice nurses.

Medical interventions can only be ordered by a GP, but limited nurse prescribing is under discussion.

Hospital and community nursing There are liaison nurses in many hospitals assigned to maintaining relations between hospital and district nursing. Liaison health visitors also exist, but they usually work in the community.

153

Funding The system of funding is going to change, introducing an internal market for health care providers. The results of this change will vary locally.

Other problems Most of the nurses who were visited in their day to day practice, reported a lack of responsibility among their patients for their own health. The generation of patients that grew up with the National Health Service in particular seems to feel that the NHS is responsible for their health, not them.

References

Baker, G., J.M. Bevan, L. Mcdonnell and B. Wall (1987), *Community Nursing; Research and Recent Developments*, Croom Helm, New York.

Butterworth, C.A. (1992), *The Nurse Practitioner in the United Kingdom*, Accepted for publication in the Journal of the Academy of Nurse Practitioners.

Crombie, D.L., P. Backer, J. Van Der Zee (1990), *The Interface Study*, EGPRW, Birmingham.

Cumberlege, J. A. Carr, P. Farmer, E. Gillepsie (1986), *Neighbourhood Nursing: A Focus for Care*, Report of the Community Nursing Review Team, Her Majesty's Stationery Office, London.

Department of Health (1990), *Report on the Advisory Group on Nurse Prescribing*, London.

Department of Health (1990), *Health and Personal Services Statistics for England 1989*, Government Statistical Service, London.

Dunnell, K. J. Dobss (1982), *Nurses Working in the Community; A survey carried out on behalf of the Department of Health and Social Security in England and Wales in 1980*, Her Majesty's Stationery Office, London.

English National Board for Nursing, Midwifery and Health Visiting (1991), *Annual report 1989-1990*, Sheffield.

Eurostat (1988), *Demographic Statistics 1988*, Luxembourg: Office des publications officielles de Communautés européennes.

Fatchett, A.B. (1990), 'Health visiting: a withering profession?' *Journal of Advanced Nursing* 15, pp. 216-222.

Findlay, M., A. Leonard, D. Mawson, A. Rothwell, S. Stenhouse, S. Rogers (1986), *Focus on District Nursing; A study of the District Nursing Service of the Wycombe Health Authority*, Wycombe Health Authority and Oxford, Regional Health Authority, Wycombe.

HMSO (1987), *Promoting better health*, HMSO, London.

Hoad, P. (1987), *The role of sociology in the teaching of post-registration nurses in Britain*, Lecture at the Tenth International Conference on Social Science and Medicine.

Kerkstra, A. (1991), 'Allround, gedifferentieerd of gespecialiseerd: lessen uit het buitenland', *Maatschappelijke Gezondheidszorg*, 19, 2, pp. 24-28.

North West Thames Regional Health Authority (1991), *Nursing in the community*, report of the working group.

OECD (1987), *Financing and Delivering Health Care; a comparative analysis of OECD countries*, Organisation for Economic Co-operation and Development, Paris.

OECD (1985), *Measuring Health Care 1960-1983; expenditure, costs and performance*, Organisation for Economic Co-operation and Development, Paris.

OECD (1988), *Ageing populations; the social policy implications*, Organisation for Economic cooperation and development, Paris.

Rawlings, M. (1991) Prescription for success, *Community outlook*, March, pp. 36-37.

Ross, F. (1985), 'A challenging district', *Nursing Mirror*, 180, 8, pp. 35-37.

Ross, F. (1987), 'District Nursing', *Recent Advances in Nursing*, 15, pp. 132-160.

Slater J. (1987), 'Health for all', *Journal of District Nursing*, 6, 4, pp. 18-22.

Smith, F. (1991), 'Pharmacists and the health care team', *Community outlook*, february, pp. 33-34.

Statistical Yearbook of Norway 1990 (1990), Statistisk Sentralbyrå, Oslo-Kongsvingen.

White, E. (1990), *Community Psychiatric Nursing*, the 1990 National Survey, Community Psychiatric Nurses Association Publications, Stockport.

WHO (1981), *Legislation Concerning Nursing/Midwifery Services and Education*, Report on a WHO study, World Health Organization, Regional Office for Europe, Copenhagen.

1. Co-author of this paragraph is drs. P. van der Heijden.

2. Main sources:
   - P.P. Groenewegen, R. Willemsen (1987), *Naar een sterkere eerste lijn? 2: Buitenlandse ervaringen*, NIVEL, Utrecht.
   - A. Maynard (1986), 'Financing the U.K. national health services', *Health Policy*, 6, 4, p. 329-340.
   - 'Minister to end discussions on GPs' new contract this month' (1989), *British Medical Journal*, 298, 6673, p. 606.
   - Department of Health (1990), *Health and personal services statistics for England*, 1990 edition, HMSO, Chapter 3, London.
   - Office of Health Economics (1989), Compendium of health statistics, OHE, Chapter 3, London.
   - E. Carrillo et al (1989), *Requirements & constraints for minimum data sets*, McAce, S.L.
   - D.L. Crombie et al (1990), *The interface study*, The Royal College of General Practitioners, London.
   - B. Abel-Smith, *Eurocare: European health care analyis*, Heath-Econ, s.a., Basle.

3. Sources: Statistical Yearbook of Norway (1990); OECD (1988).

4. Source: Crombie et al (1990).

5. In July 1992 a majority of English dentists have decided not to accept any more adult patients on the NHS. They will continue to see existing patients, but these patients will have to pay higher fees, almost as in private medicine.
   The reason for this is a dispute over funding between the government and dentists.

9 Community nursing in the United States

The setting

Population

* total population (1987)   243,8 million
* % over 65 (1987)   12,3
* % over 65 (2000, projected)   12,2
* % over 65 (2010, projected)   12,8
* % over 65 (2020, projected)   16,2
* % under 15 (1987)   21,5
* life expectancy at birth (years)(1985)   71,2 (men)
                                                           79,0 (women)
* live births per 1000 inhabitants (1988)   15,9
* population density per sq. kilometre (1987)   26
* population groups: many large population groups. Besides European immigrants who came in the 19th and the first half of the 20th century, there is a large minority from Middle and South America (Sources: Statistical Yearbook of Norway (1990), OECD (1988)).

Health care system

Introduction The USA is a federal union with considerable decision making powers delegated to states, counties, and communities. Furthermore, the laissez-faire policy has resulted in a highly pluralistic organization of health care.

Roemer (1986) discerns governmental departments of health and human services at state and national levels, which shape the legal limitations within which the health care system has to operate. Besides these there is a great variety of other government agencies, for-profit and non-profit organizations.

159

Health insurance   There are two public insurance schemes: Medicare and Medicaid.

Medicare is the Federal insurance scheme designed for the elderly population. Medicaid is a public insurance scheme financed by Federal and State governments (see 9.2.2).

There is an enormous series of voluntary health insurances. First of all there are the commercial insurance companies, second, the non-profit Blue Cross and Blue Shield organizations and third, the Prepaid Health Plans.

About 12% of the population is neither covered by public nor by voluntary health insurance (Roemer, 1986). More recent census data of the department of health and human services give an even higher percentage (13.1%) (Source: questionnaire).

Funding

Table 9.1
Total and public expenditure on health care in the USA

year	total expend. % GDP	public expend. % GDP	expend. in US $ per head
1980	9.23	3.91	1089
1981	9.54	4.03	1247
1982	10.37	4.33	1392
1983	10.65	4.40	1521
1984	10.44	4.29	1639
1985	10.56	4.41	1751
1986	10.87	4.51	1886
1987	11.19	4.63	2051

Source: Programme ECO-SANTE, BASYS/CREDES

Ambulatory medical care   It has to be noted that the European concept of General Practitioners (or Family Physicians) is not very well known in the US. Most physicians are specialists, of whom many are working office based (as opposed to hospital based). General Practitioners do not have a gate-keeper role for specialist care except in Prepaid Health Plans like Health Maintenance Organizations or Preferred Provider Organizations. In these plans there is increased emphasis and funding for primary care providers.

Patients usually do not register with a GP. Patients are free to choose the physician they want. If a patient is taking part in a Prepaid Health Plan, like a Health Maintenance Organization or a Preferred Provider Organization, however, the choice is limited.

Institutional care There are public as well as private hospitals. The mean length of stay in somatic hospitals in days (1980) was 13.3 (OECD, 1987).

Table 9.2
Inpatient medical care beds and personnel per bed

year	beds total	beds per 1000	personnel per bed
1980	1364500	6.0	2.56
1981	1361500	5.9	2.69
1982	1359800	5.8	2.91
1983	1350400	5.8	2.75
1984	1338700	5.6	2.71
1985	1308500	5.5	2.77
1986	1283000	5.3	2.84
1987	1267000	5.2	2.95

Source: Programme ECO-SANTE, BASYS/CREDES

Community nursing

In the United States there are various types of organizations for home care which all originate from public health nursing. Public health nursing organizations cared about public health in the broadest sense of the word in a community. Today Public Health Nursing refers to mainly preventive activities in the community as a whole (as opposed to the individual client).

The term Community Nursing was invented for those types of nursing of which the main concern was to care for individual patients or families. The following terms refer to various types of community nursing.
- Home Health Care (general care at home)
- Hospice Care (for terminal illness)
- Ambulatory Care (outpatient care)
- School Care
- Occupational Care (care organised by employers)

A special type of community nursing is provided by nurse practitioners, who have masters degrees in nursing. Most nurse practitioners work independently, often reimbursed by governments and often from an ambulatory care setting. Often a patient's first contact with health care is initiated through a nurse practitioner. She is allowed to do physical examinations, assesses a patient's health history, refers to other care providers, does some limited prescription.

In the following emphasis will be placed on home health care. In home health care we will concentrate on two types of organizations that come closest to the definition of organizations to be taken into account that was given in the introduction.

- Visiting Nurses Associations/Agencies
- Home Health Agencies

There are no principal differences between these types of organizations.

Among Home Health Agencies / Visiting Nurse Associations three distinctions are made.

1   Between
     - Medicare-certified home health agencies and
     - non-Medicare home health agencies
     As of February 1990 there were 5701 Medicare-certified agencies and 5500 non-Medicare home health agencies in the United States (National Association for Home Care, 1991).
2   Between private organizations and public organizations.
3   Between non-profit and for-profit organizations. The for-profit sector is rapidly developing (Shuster, 1991).

The following description of home health care in the United States will largely be based on questionnaires from two Medicare-certified, non-profit, private visiting nurse services.

1   V(isiting) N(urse) S(ervice) Home Care in New York (VNSNY)
2   Visiting Nurse Association of Greater Philadelphia

Though all organizations provide a variety of services the following will be concentrated on the various types of nursing services.

History

General   According to Smith (1989) socio-cultural trends like urbanization and an increasing influx of immigrants and health problems in the United States have historically shaped public health nursing, the precursor to community health nursing. The emphasis in public health nursing was on preventive care and the creation of a healthy and more sanitary environment. In the second half of this century medical advancements made this type of work less important and the emphasis shifted towards a more individually oriented type of care. This shift was enhanced by the 1965 Amendments of the Social Security Act of 1935, that introduced a new vision on government sponsorship of health care services in the form of the Medicare legislation. The rights of the elderly and poor population started to resemble more those of the privately insured population. The trade-off has been the loss of a continuum of preventive and health promotion services that were provided

162

through the public health system.

In the early 1980s diagnosis related groups (DRGs) were introduced in funding hospital care. For each type of diagnosis of a fixed amount of money per patient was paid to hospitals. A logical consequence of this is that hospitals are very concerned with shortening the length of stay of patients, and thereby creating a greater demand for aftercare at home. The average length of stay has declined from 10.3 days in 1981 (before DRGS) to 8.8 days by 1984 (after DRGS) (Shuster, 1991).

Visiting Nurse Service of New York (VNSNY) The Visiting Nurses Service of New York was the first secular based home nursing service, established by Lillian Wald (in 1893) who was one of the pioneers of home nursing in the USA. The purpose of this organization was to provide health services to the city's poor. The organization extended its services during the 20th century, providing not only nursing care but also social work and home health aide.

In 1986 the service was confronted with federal government reductions in spending on Medicare and between 1984 and 1988 eligibility requirements for Medicare became much stricter, leading to an increase in retrospective denials of payment (see Harris, 1988b). The result of this was to focus on more cost efficient payers and form alternative reimbursement strategies. In 1986, a joint venture was organized between the non-profit sector within VNSNY and the for-profit sector to create some budgetary space.

Visiting Nurse Association of Greater Philadelphia (VNAGP) The VNAGP started by the end of the 19th century as an organization for preventive mother and child care, teaching health care to mothers with babies to reduce infant mortality. It developed into an organization delivering all kinds of nursing care including, since 1991, rehabilitation care and home health aid.

Organization and funding

Funding According to Buhler-Wilkerson (1989) government sponsored home care services are primarily funded through the federal Medicare program. Additional federal programs (like Medicaid), however, do exist, subsidizing non-privately insured individuals to purchase home care services in the private market.

The most important sources of income for the VNSNY as well as VNAGP are Medicare and Medicaid (Table 9.3). Additional sources of finance for the VNAGP consist of funds raised in the community from private and corporate grants.

163

Table 9.3

Visiting Nurse Services of New York's payer mix for 1990 and Visiting Nurse Association of Greater Philadelphia's 1990 sources of income

	VNSNY	VNAGP	
Medicare	39%	-	
			85%
Medicaid	46%	-	
Blue Cross private insurance	5%	-	
			5%
other private insurance	8%	-	
private Pay and Free (charity) Care	2%	2%	
funds raised in the community	-	7%	

Source: questionnaire VNSNY, questionnaire VNAGP

The purpose of *Medicaid* insurance is to provide payment for a comprehensive range of medical services for persons with low income and resources. Medicaid is a partnership between state and federal government and there are considerable differences between states. Applicants for Medicaid must qualify as 'medically needy individuals' according to the following medical requirements:
- the patient's medical condition must be stable;
- the patient's health and safety in the home can be adequately assured with the provision of home services;
- the service must be requested by a physician.

All home care services require authorization in advance though it often happens that authorization takes place after the first visits have taken place. Financial eligibility is based on monthly income limits and poverty levels. If a patient's income and resources is more than the amount specified by Medicaid, he/she is responsible for paying this overhead on a monthly basis regardless of the cost of the services. According to the January 1990 income and resource levels in New York state, if a family size of 3 had a monthly income of USD 709.- and resources equal to USD 5750.- then no extra payment was required. If that family's income was USD 800.- then USD 91.- was required, irrespective of the services delivered.

Medicare was intended to increase access to health care service and to reduce the financial burden of the high costs of medical care for the elderly. It is funded by the federal government.

The conditions for recipients of Home Health Services under Medicare include:
- beneficiary must be confined to his home;

- beneficiary needs skilled nursing care or physical or speech therapy (custodial care is not covered)
- skilled care must be needed on an intermittent basis (part-time, not on a continuous basis);
- services are rendered in accordance with a plan established and reviewed by physician;
- services are furnished while beneficiary is under the care of a physician.

It should be noted here that Medicare employs the same conditions for eligibility for nursing and home health aide services.

If a Medicare recipient meets the above conditions, he/she is theoretically entitled to an unlimited number of home health visits. However, this rarely happens because of Medicare's policy of strictly interpreting conditions for coverage.

Specific items not covered under Medicare include certain medical equipment (i.e. bathroom safety equipment) supplies (i.e. diapers), drugs (infusion therapy solutions) and custodial care. There is a voluntary option for a supplementary medical insurance program that requires a monthly premium (USD 30,- as of March 1991). Under this coverage, Medicare reimburses 80% of its 'allowed charges' on home health services, medical equipment and supplies. Medicare defines 'allowed charges' as the lowest or customary charge (Source: questionnaire VNSNY).

The nurses are paid directly from the certified service on a fee for service basis or salary. The nurses incomes in VNSNY are indicated below.

Licensed practical nurse	$ 24 per visit or yearly $ 19,000 - $ 32,000
Public health nurse	$ 41-43 per visit or yearly $ 37,500 - $ 54,000
Professional nurse	same
NOVA nurse	same
Paediatric nurse	same
Mental health/ psychiatric nurse	same

Source: questionnaire VNSNY

Organizational requirements for Medicare certified agencies The State Department of Health in New York state is responsible for establishing regulatory standards, legislative policies and general oversight of certified agencies.

The regulatory standards for Medicare certified agencies are listed below.

A   Two-thirds of nursing service have to be provided directly by the admitting agency; they can not be subcontracted to other agencies.

B   Nursing and home health aide services have to be available 24 hours a day, seven days a week;

C   Agencies have to initiate patient care, where appropriate, within 24 hours after referral;

D Medicare certified organizations are responsible for ensuring that all subcontracted services are provided by agencies that are not only licensed by the state but in compliance with licensure requirements.

E A patient grievance or complaint procedure has to be established.

F Agencies have to thoroughly document reasons for discharge. Agencies can discharge a patient only if he or she required a different level of medical care or if the patient terminated services.

In addition, applicants for certification also have to ensure access to and quality of care, admit all eligible patients within the entire planning area regardless of case complexity, place of residence, race, age, or payment source, and provide charity care (= free care, see Table 9.3) that equals no less than 2 percent of projected total annual operating costs.

The certified agencies themselves co-ordinate, monitor and provide actual services by employing nurses and other health care professionals.

Organization of the Visiting Nurse Service of New York Within the organization a distinction is made between various programs for various types of patients and problems for which we refer to page 171/172.

The Visiting Nurse Service of New York has to compete with other Certified Home Health agencies in the New York City area (approximately 44 agencies).

Expert knowledge is available within the organization. The organization initiates training programs for identified knowledge gaps and/or patterns of problems in the service. Inservice programs are provided by both internal specialist nurses and public training groups. To co-ordinate these programs a special Educational Director is appointed.

The Visiting Nurses Association operates from borough offices. All types of personnel listed in Table 9.6 work in these borough offices in the numbers depending on the needs of the borough. The boroughs are divided into communities and within those communities patients are usually seen by the same nurse.

Organization of the Visiting Nurse Association of Greater Philadelphia The VNAGP is a much smaller organization though it covers an area of about 400,000 inhabitants. Within the organization a distinction is made between

1 Acute care, providing skilled nursing care on an intermittent basis to patients in acute stages or terminal illness.

2 Private duty care providing shifts up to 24 hours a day of nursing, home health aid or homemaker assistance to acutely or chronically ill patients.

3 Preventive Programs providing health teaching to mothers of high risk pregnancy or premature infants and providing communicable disease follow-up care often by contract with government agencies.

Expert knowledge is available within the organization from nutritionists and nurse clinicians who are specialised in wound care, infusion care, geriatrics and psychiatry.

The organization has to compete with for-profit organizations, hospital based home health companies and other visiting nurse agencies.

Nurses are paid a salary, though visits made after normal working hours at the weekend may be paid at a visit rate in addition to the salary.

Patients are not seen on site but only visited at home, so there is only a need for office space for nurses and administration.

The organization can be reached 24 hours a day (this is one of the conditions for Medicare-certification) and care can be delivered 24 hours a day if necessary.

Nurses work in teams which cover a geographic area. Mother and child health nurses, however work solo, taking personal care of an area.

Types of community nurses and manpower

Education Towards the end of the nineteenth century nursing was introduced as a discipline with formal training. Educational programs were generally only available in hospitals. The Goldmark report, published in 1923 showed that many of these hospital-based schools were not able to provide adequate educational facilities and it recommended the training of nurses be placed under the control of colleges and universities. However, in 1952, 92 percent of all graduations from pre-licensure RN schools of nursing still took place at hospital-based schools and it took another 30 years for this figure to drop to 15 percent (1982). Hospital schools are gradually affiliating with universities of colleges (Roemer, 1986).

We can distinguish 5 professions concerned with nursing in the United States:

Registered Nurses (RNs), who are licensed by the state after having graduated from highschool and who have taken one of the following: a hospital-based diploma program, or a college; university-based program; a university-based baccalaureate program or a junior college-based associate degree program. Advanced training is available in the form of college- or university-based master's and doctoral programs. According to Moses (1990) a significant change has occurred in the distribution of the registered nurse population in terms of the type of basic training taken to qualify as a registered nurse. 10 Years earlier, three-quarters of nurses had received their initial educational preparation in a hospital based diploma program. In 1988 slightly less than half of the nurses had graduated from such programs. Among those who had graduated within the last fifteen years, only 22 percent were diploma school graduates. Figures for the total 1988 nurse population in community or public health are presented in Table 9.4. In addition to the highest level of nursing training listed below about 78% of the total number of nurses employed had taken short term courses during the previous year.

Table 9.4
Employed registered nurse population in community or public health setting in 1988 by highest nursing related training (N=110,886)

diploma	31%
associate Degree	21%
baccalaureate	37%
master's degree	10%
doctorate	0.1%

Source: Moses, 1990

It will be clear from Table 9.4 that the term 'Registered Nurse' includes different levels of education.

Licensed Practical Nurses (LPNs) have completed a one year program after highschool (Roemer, 1986).

Nurse's aides, orderlies, home health aides, and attendants have usually had on-the-job training sometimes with a short formal training program. (Roemer, 1986).

General manpower According to Moses (1990) 6.8 percent or 110,886 of the total number of registered nurses were employed in community or public health settings. This number accounts for a nurse-population ratio of one community/public health nurse for every 2,217 inhabitants. It should be remembered, however, that this figure only includes registered nurses and does not refer to the total nursing workforce.

Manpower of the Visiting Nurse Services of New York Table 9.5 gives the number of nurses in New York State.

Table 9.5
Absolute number or nurses and number of inhabitants per nurse in New York state in 1989 (nurses working for Medicare certified agencies only)

	no. of nurses	nurse: population ratio
public health and professional nurses	3,500	5,117
licensed practical nurses	100	179,090

Source: questionnaire VNSNY

The Visiting Nurse Service of New York accounts for a large part of the total number of nurses in New York State. Table 9.6 gives the number of various types of personnel in VNSNY. Most striking is the low figure for licensed practical nurses and the large total work force.

Table 9.6
Personnel employed by the Visiting Nurse Service of New York (full-time equivalents)

non-nursing staff	
physical therapists	150
occupational therapists	75
speech therapists	48
nutritional consultants	12
social workers	164
volunteers	250
subtotal	*699*

nursing staff	
public health nurses*	415
registered nurses*	475
licensed practical nurses	25
NOVA nurses (see 'types of care')*	20
pediatric nurses	1
psychiatric nurses	8
subtotal	*944*

total	1632

*   The VNSNY employs the following definitions:
-   Public Health Nurse: bachelors of Science in Nursing (4 years at a university)
-   Registered Nurse: Associates Degree in Nursing (2 years at a university) plus one year experience.
-   NOVA nurses: Bachelor of Science and NOVA certificate
-   Paediatric nurse: Associates degree in Nursing plus one year experience.
-   Licensed practical nurse: Associates degree in nursing

These requirements are flexible in that training may be substituted for experience.

Source: questionnaire VNSNY

Manpower Visiting Nurse Association of Greater Philadelphia The VNAGP is a much smaller organization than the VNSNY. Table 9.7 shows the various types of personnel employed by VNAGP.

Table 9.7
Personnel employed by VNAGP in full-time equivalents

non-nursingstaff

physical therapists	25
occupational therapists	3
speech therapists	2
social workers	4.5
home health aides	67

advanced practice nurses:

medical/surgical specialist nurses	1
psychiatric specialist nurses	1
infusion care specialist nurses	1

general nursingstaff:

maternal/child health nurses	6
medical/surgical adult nurses	80

The advanced practice nurses are clinical specialists with a masters degree in nursing or a diploma in nursing or a bachelors degree in nursing, combined with a specialty course of 12 months in stoma/wound care, maternal/child health care or other specialty. The general nursing staff has a diploma or a bachelors degree in nursing. Licensed practical nurses are not employed by the VNAGP.

Because the VNAGP is not the only organization serving the area, it is impossible to give nurse-population ratio's.

Patient populations

Visiting Nurse Service of New York

Table 9.8
Patient characteristics VNSNY clients

age		percentage of clients according to program (see 1.2.4)	
0-5	12.5%		
6-20	5.7%	adult care patients	65%
21-45	14.6%	maternal/child health	22%
46-65	15.8%	paediatrics	8%
66-75	17.8%	AIDS patients	2%
76-90	29.8%	hospice patients	1%
91+	3.8%	long term care	1%
		infusion therapy care	1%

Source: questionnaire VNSNY

More than 50% of all patients are over 65. Of course this figure is reflected in the number of patients in adult care (65%)

Visiting Nurse Association of Greater Philadelphia More than 90% of the total client population are over 60, and about 80% are receiving post-operative and aftercare (Table 9.9)

Table 9.9

Patient characteristics VNAGP clients

age		reason for care	
under 5	5%	pregnancies	1%
5-19	2.5%	mothers and newborns	2%
20-59	2.5%	mentally handicapped	1%
60-79	80%	physically handic.	5%
over 80	10%	mentally ill	1%
		terminally ill	5%
		chronically ill	5%
		post-operative/aftercare	80%

Source: questionnaire VNAGP

Types of care

Visiting Nurse Service of New York VNSNY provides various programs of care, some of which are typical for a large city like New York.

A   Programs to alleviate overcrowding in hospitals:

- *Home Health Intake Program* employing Home Health Intake Co-ordinators in 20 hospitals in the city who facilitate discharge planning and maintain continuity of home care.
- *Preferred Provider Program* in which VNSNY participates as the preferred provider of home care services.
- *Early Maternity Discharge Program* through which mothers with normal deliveries can shorten the length of stay in maternity hospitals. VNSNY monitors the health of mother and child, provides reassurance, clarifies questions about infant care, and instructs other family members in the baby's care.

B   A program for terminally ill to enable them to spend the remaining time they have in their own homes: *The Hospice Program*. Hospice coverage under Medicare has a life-time limitation of two periods of 90 days and a subsequent period of 30 days, each period requiring certification. Each Medicare certified organization has a fixed number of places for hospice patients.

C   Programs to address the growing number of the elderly with chronic illnesses:

- *Adult Care Program* provides short- and longterm medical nursing, supportive services, and rehabilitation therapy.
- *Partners in Care* is a supportive service for elderly who are unable to co-ordinate the care themselves but who wish to pay for the home care ser-

vices themselves. Partners in Care assesses the needs of the applicant and co-ordinates the care either from VNS programs or other community services.

- *Meals on Wheels*.
- *Telephone Reassurance Program*. This program is run by volunteers and is particularly important for the elderly who often need reminders to take their medication and to keep doctor's appointments.
- *The Long Term Home Health Care Program*: the Lombardi Program which focuses on improving the quality of life for clients who are able to remain at home by providing for instance heavy duty cleaning and social transportation.

D   Programs to address the poor health status of infants and children.

- *The Maternal/Child Health and Paediatric Program* sends nurses, developmental specialists, therapists and social workers to work with impoverished children and their families.
- *The FIRST STEPS Program* to address the problems of drug-abusing women in their child bearing years.
- *Paediatric Respite Program* supporting families caring for a chronically ill or severely disabled child at home.

E   *AIDS services*, providing an organizing various types of care for AIDS or HIV positive patients.

F   *Community Mental Health Services*.

G   NOVA: *Nutrition Oncology and Vascular Access*. This program provides advanced medical therapies such as total parenteral nutrition, hydration, antibiotic, continuous pain control and select chemotherapy.

Source: Visiting Nurse Service of New York, 1990

Nurses in the VNSNY are in most cases specialized in one of the services mentioned above.

The percentages of the total working time spent on selected activities is shown in Table 9.10 for the types of VNSNY nurses indicated in Table 9.6. The licensed practical nurses are less concerned with paperwork and more with home visiting than the other nurses.

Table 9.10
Percentage of time spent on selected activities by VNSNY nurses (estimates)

	public health nurses registered nurses paediatric nurses mental health nurses	licensed practical nurses
home visits	66%	75%
all preventive activities	50%	50%
administration/paperwork	33%	25%

Source: questionnaire VNSNY

Besides the differences listed above, the licensed practical nurses do not perform the more complicated technical nursing procedures.

Visiting Nurse Association of Greater Philadelphia The VNAGP does not have such an extended list of programs as the VNSNY has. This organization is less organizationally specialized but offers, generally speaking, the same services. Care is only provided in the homes of patients and therefore nurses spend most of their working time on home visits (Table 9.11)

Table 9.11
Time spent on selected activities by VNAGP nurses (estimates)

	home visits hours*	con- sultation	paper- work
medical/surgical specialists	30%	30%	25%
psychiatric specialists	30%	30%	25%
infusion care specialists	30%	5%	25%
mother and child health care specialists	80%	-	25%
medical/surgical generalists	80%	-	25%

* consultation hours for other staff, not for clients.

Source: questionnaire VNAGP

Visiting Nurse Service of New York Referrals for home health care services are categorized in Table 9.12.

Table 9.12
Referrals for home health care of the VNSNY

hospitals	69%
physicians	5%
adult homes / shelters	10%
self/ community	16%

Source: questionnaire VNSNY

The high percentage of referrals from hospitals comes from the VNSNY staff placed in hospitals and from hospital social work / discharge planners. After referral assessment is done by a public health or professional nurse who also assesses the possible need for home help care. Assessment is done using standardized forms. Assessment should be done, however, in conjunction with a physician.

Nurse supervisors in the previously mentioned boroughs decide who is going to deliver the care. Once this is done a patient service manual comes into force that quite exactly determines what is done in what stage of the care delivery by whom. Evaluation takes place at a minimum of every 60 days based upon patient's needs. The physician's orders have to be renewed every 62 days.

Visiting Nurse Association of Greater Philadelphia Referrals for home health care services are categorized in Table 9.13.

Table 9.13
Referrals for home health care for VNAGP

patient's family	2.5%
patient him/herself	2.5%
home help services	5%
hospital or nursing home for elderly	80%
other prof. careproviders (e.g. physicians)	10%

Source: questionnaire VNAGP

175

Assessment is done by any kind of therapist or nurse listed in Table 9.7. He or she may also assess the need for home health aide services and determines who is going to deliver the care. No check lists for assessment are used, contrary to VNSNY and many other organizations (see for instance Jaffe and Skidmore-Roth, 1988; Jackson and Neighbors, 1990).

In general the professional who delivers the care is responsible for his own actions. The nurse or therapist is responsible for errors in actions of the home health aide only if he or she instructed that aide to carry out an unsafe procedure. The same is true of the responsibility of the physician for ordering a harmful procedure or medication.

Evaluation of care takes place regularly. At least quarterly a sample of records is reviewed. If a specific type of problem is identified, monthly samples may be taken until the type of error is corrected. Besides this, one of the requirements of Medicare is that authorization must be renewed every two months, so that each two months the situation is evaluated, at least by a physician.

An interesting study worth mentioning here took place at the *Visiting Nurse Association of Eastern Montgomery County*. In this study patients were classified into 5 groups (Recovery, Self Care, Rehabilitation, Maintenance and Terminal). For each group goals were formulated and the level of attainment of these goals was related to the amount of time spent on each patient (Harris et al., 1988).

Relations with general practitioners, home help services and hospitals

Visiting Nurse Services of New York Nurses have to co-operate with physicians throughout the patient's period of care (this is one of the Medicare requirements) and hospital social workers during patient discharge. They have to co-operate with other health care personnel (physical therapists, home health aides, etc.) for the co-ordination and management of care. Some of the programs listed in 9.2.4 specifically refer to co-operation and co-ordination, also with hospitals.

There are at least 15 agencies in New York city that can provide different levels of home help, varying from Home health aide (which is the highest level of home help care i.e. simple dressings, assistance with rehabilitation therapy) to home attendant (light housekeeping, meal preparation, etc.).

The nurses may have to deal with a large number of physicians.

Visiting Nurse Association of Greater Philadelphia The VNAGP nurses and therapists co-operate with hospital discharge planners and other therapists serving the same patient. Since Medicare requires authorization of a physician, they also have to co-operate with these. The number of General Practitioners that a nurse has to deal with may be up to 50. In general the nurses only have to deal with 2 home help services.

Relations with hospitals are maintained through liaison nurses in the hospital. She meets the patient in the hospital and, through discussion with the hospital nurses, the physician and the patient, plans the home care referral.

Problems

Underperformance Activities that were considered underperformed consisted of the following:
Hygienic and other personal care, psychosocial activities, encouragement of help from family members and home help care for elderly patients.

Other reported underperformed activities concerned mainly the publicly insured who seemed to be in need of more nursing care of any type. Furthermore, assessment of groups at risk seemed to be a considerable problem as well as the provision of information on medicine, diet and nutrition.

Personnel shortages There appears to be a nationwide shortage of community nurses.

In New York City the shortage of community nurses can be attributed to the working environment, which may include working in unsafe neighbourhoods, length of commuting to work, cost of living in the area, patient population and amount of reimbursement. Reimbursement in hospitals is higher than in the community. Harris (1990) describes some of the problems in home care that make the work less attractive for nurses and that endanger the quality of care. She mentions for instance the fact that promotive activities are non-reimbursable in most cases; the pressure on staff to maintain a high number of visits, in spite of fluctuating caseloads, which is due to the system of reimbursement per visit; the shortage of personnel; increasing use of risk taking high-tech possibilities with liability consequences which calls for more expertise on legal issues.

Specialist versus generalist Nurses in the VNSNY are in most cases working in the specific care programs that were mentioned in above. No problems were reported concerning this method of working.

In the VNAGP there is less specialization, but here too no problems were reported.

Levels of experience and home helps No problems were reported in respect of the division of tasks among different types of nurses. It has to be noted that in both organizations there are hardly any second level (licenced practical) nurses.

Home helps are not represented in the VNSNY. In New York different levels of home help are often provided by for-profit organizations. In the VNAGP home help services are integrated. No problems were reported by the VNAGP, nor by the VNSNY.

Community nursing and general practitioner/physician
For Medicare and Medicaid patients it is necessary that the services are requested by and take place in accordance with a physician. Authorization needs to be periodically renewed by a physician.

Hospital and community nursing In the early nineteen eighties Diagnostic Related Groups (DRGs) were introduced in the funding of hospitals. This made it financially more attractive for hospitals to discharge patients earlier. It created a greater demand for home nursing.

In about 20 hospitals in New York there are home health intake co-ordinators employed by the VNSNY to facilitate discharge planning and maintain continuity of home care. In other hospitals there may be liaison nurses.

No problems were reported on this issue.

Funding Long-term care in the home is being threatened by lack of funding. Currently, the poor usually can receive this type of care but this may change because of Medicaid regulations that become more strict. The alternative will be placement in nursing homes with strict financial requirements. The VNAGP questionnaire adds that Medicaid provides only a very limited amount of home care in that state and that therefore the agency is very much dependent on donated funds from private or corporate donors.

Other problems There is some discussion on case management. In a White Paper by the Government Affairs Committee (1991) the division of tasks between various care providers and funding bodies is discussed.

References

Buhler-Wilkerson, K. (1989), *Home care the American way*, Paper presented at the International Conference on Community Nursing, 16-17 March, 's-Hertogenbosch, The Netherlands.

Government Affairs Committee (1991), *Case Management*, a white paper prepared by the government affairs committee, approved by the Board of the National Association for Home Care, January 1990, Washington.

Harris, M.D., D.A. Peters, J. Ivan (1988), *Relating quality and cost in a Home Health Care Agency*, Joint Commission on Accreditation of Health Care Organizations , Chicago.

Jackson, J.E., M. Neighbors (1990), *Home Care Client Assessment*, Handbook, Rockville, Aspen Publishers Inc., Maryland.

Jaffe, M.S., L. Skidmore-Roth (1988), *Home Health Nursing Care Plans*, The C.V. Mosby Company, St. Louis.

Moses, E.B. (1990), *The registered nurse population, findings from the National Sample Survey of Registered Nurses, March 1988*, U.S. Department of Health and Human Services, Public Health Service, Health Resources and Services Administration, Bureau of Health Professions, Division of Nursing.

National Association for Home Care (1991), Legislative Blueprint for Action.

OECD (1988), *Ageing populations; the social policy implications*, Organization for economic co-operation and development, Paris.

Roemer, M.I. (1986), *An Introduction to the U.S. Health Care System* (second edition), Springer Publishing Company Inc., New York.

Shuster, G.F. and P.A. Cloonan (1991), 'Home Health Nursing Care: A comparison of not-for-profit and for-profit agencies', *Home Health Care Services Review Quarterly*, 12, 1.

Smith, G.R. (1989), *Community Health nursing in the United States*, In: A. Kerkstra and R. Verheij: Community Nursing, Proceedings of the International Conference on community Nursing, 16-17 March 1989, 's-Hertogenbosch, The Netherlands, Netherlands Institute of Primary Health Care, Utrecht.

Statistical Yearbook of Norway 1990 (1990), Statistisk Sentralbyrå, Oslo-Kongsvingen.

Visiting Nurse Service of New York (1990), *Annual report 1989*, New York.

10 Summary and conclusions

Introduction

In the preceding chapters the functioning, funding and organization of community nursing in nine different countries was described. In the present chapter an attempt will be made to compare the countries on some of the issues. In doing this the situation in each country is generalized, sometimes neglecting important exceptions. In order not to confuse the reader too much, only those organizations are taken into account in this chapter that deliver adult and elderly care, leaving out those organizations that have specialised in child health care.

The general lines will be followed according to which the countries were described.

The setting

Population

One of the most important determinants of the need for home care is the percentage of the population above 65 years of age (Table 10.1).

All countries reported the growing number of the elderly being of great concern regarding the future need for community care. It appears from the table, however, that the countries show quite a lot of variation in the percentage of the population above 65 years of age, and the pace at which this percentage is growing. Germany in particular will face a very large proportion of elderly in the coming decades.

Table 10.1
Percentage of population over 65 in nine countries, 1987, 2000, 2010, 2020, 2030, 2040, 2050 (projected)

	1987	2000	2010	2020	2030	2040	2050
Norway	16.2	15.2	15.1	18.2	20.7	22.8	21.9
UK	15.3	14.5	14.6	16.3	19.2	20.4	18.7
Germany	15.1	17.1	20.4	21.7	25.8	27.6	24.5
Belgium	14.3	14.7	15.9	17.7	20.8	21.9	20.8
France	13.8	15.3	16.3	19.5	21.8	22.7	22.3
Finland	13.1	14.4	16.8	21.7	23.8	23.1	22.7
Netherlands	12.5	13.5	15.1	18.9	23.0	24.8	22.6
USA	12.3	12.2	12.8	16.2	19.5	19.8	19.3
Canada	10.7	12.8	14.6	18.6	22.4	22.5	21.3

Sources: Statistical Yearbook of Norway, 1990, OECD 1988

Health care system

The most important differences in the health insurance systems are given below.

Norway:	One national system
Finland:	One national system
England:	One national system
Canada:	One national system
Netherlands:	AWBZ (national system)
	Public insurance
	Private insurance above certain income levels
France:	Various public insurance schemes with
	Options for additional insurance
Belgium:	Public insurance for employees
	Public insurance for self-employed
	Options for additional insurance
Germany:	Public insurance and
	Private insurance above certain income levels
USA:	Medicare and Medicaid
	Private insurance or no insurance for all others

It should be remembered that there may be considerable differences between public health insurance schemes. In France and Germany for example there can be considerable differences between the various health insurance funds which operate the public health scheme. Of course the same is true for the national health insurance schemes.

Funding There are considerable differences in expenditure on health care among the nine countries (Table 10.2). Especially the United States have a very high total expenditure on health care, combined with a very low public expenditure. The cheapest system appears to be the NHS in the United Kingdom.

Table 10.2
Total expenditure and public expenditure on health care as percentage of GDP in nine countries

	total expend. % of GDP	public expend. % of GDP
Belgium	7.45	5.73
Canada	8.69	6.42
UK	6.05	5.23
Finland	7.4	5.8
France	8.52	6.37
Germany	8.06	6.33
Netherlands	8.46	6.25
Norway	7.5	7.4
USA	11.19	4.63

Source: Program ECO-SANTE by BASYS and CREDES

Community nursing

History

In many countries community nursing has a religious background. For example, in Germany this can still be seen from the system of umbrella organizations with each its own religious affiliation.
In both Scandinavian countries a religious background is not known. In these countries community nursing became the responsibility of the local government in a relatively early stage.

183

In all countries the need for community nursing care became clear during the industrial revolution. Community nursing in those days was particularly concerned with preventive care for the whole population in order to fight epidemic diseases. In the second half of the twentieth century the emphasis of the activities shifted towards more individually oriented care.

Organization and funding

Organization child health care and adult/elderly care An important feature in the organization of community nursing is whether child health care and adult and elderly care are provided by the same organization. Generally speaking these two services are organized separately in Belgium, Germany, Canada and the USA, while it varies in France (Table 10.3). It should be remembered that being in the same organization does not imply that the same nurses give both types of care.

Table 10.3
Organizational separation between adult care and child health care

country	separate organizations
Belgium	yes
Canada (Ontario)	yes
England	no
Finland	no
France	varies
Germany	yes
Netherlands	no
Norway	no
USA	yes

Integration with health and social services In many countries community nursing is part of an organization that is providing other - non-nursing - health services (e.g. physiotherapy, chiropody, general medical care) and social services (e.g. social work, home help) as well. This, however, does not always mean that these other services are provided at or from the same place as community nursing care. This is an important distinction, since it is generally assumed that being in the same organization gives better possibilities for communication. The influence of working from the same premises, however, is equally important. Table 10.4 gives an overview of these features in nine countries. The table provides very general information and it should be remembered that there are exceptions in all countries.

In the preceding chapters it has already been shown that in many countries home help services and community nursing services are integrating. This is reflected in the table: England is the only country in which there is, generally speaking, no integration between the two services. In Belgium and the Netherlands there are just a few organizations combining the two services. In the Netherlands, however, integration will take place in the next few years.

Table 10.4
Organizational characteristics of community nursing in nine countries

country	non nursing health service in same organization	non nursing health services in same location	home help services in same organization	home help help services in same location
Belgium	no	no	seldomly	seldomly
Canada	some provinces	some provinces	some provinces	some provinces
England	no	often	no	no
Finland	yes	sometimes	yes	sometimes
France	?	?	sometimes	sometimes
Germany	no	no	often	often
Netherlands	no	seldomly	seldomly	seldomly
Norway	yes	often	yes	sometimes
USA	sometimes	sometimes	sometimes	sometimes

Specialist knowledge Most organizations in most countries employ specialist nurses or other professionals who are either working in the field or at a higher level in the organization. Sometimes the sources of specialist knowledge are supplemented by sources from outside the organization.

Governmental role Governmental bodies play a substantial role in the provision of community nursing care in all countries studied. But there are differences. In comparison with the Scandinavian countries for instance, in France, Germany and the USA much is left to private initiative.

185

Table 10.5
Relative importance of governmental bodies in the provision of community nursing

	low	middle	high
Belgium		x	
Canada			x
Finland			x
France	x		
Germany	x		
Netherlands			x*
Norway			x
United Kingdom			x
United States	x		

*   Cross associations are in fact private organizations but they have a monopoly position and are almost entirely funded by the government.

24-Hour accessability Another organizational characteristic discussed was 24-hour accessability by telephone (Table 10.6). Most countries appear to have a round-the-clock accessability.

Table 10.6
24-hours accessability of community nursing organizations in nine countries

Belgium	yes	
Canada (Ontario)	yes	
UK	sometimes	
Finland	yes	
France	sometimes	
Germany	sometimes	
Netherlands	yes	
Norway	in large municipalities:	yes
USA	medicare-licenced agencies:	yes

Independent Nurses In all countries there are organized services for community nursing care. This, however, does not imply that all community nursing services in all countries are organized. In France, Belgium and the USA it was reported that there is a quantitatively important group of independent nurses that may have contracts with organizations but who are in fact self employed.

Geographic assignment In most countries nurses work for a specific area. Nurses or teams of nurses, are assigned to a geographic area. Attachment to a GP seems to be a phenomenon exclusive to England though experiments are being carried out with this method of working in Finland and nurses working in health centers in the Netherlands often are GP-attached too. The difference between England and Finland in this respect is, however, that GPs in Finland work in specific areas and that the GP-attached nurses consequently do so too, whereas in England the GPs have less strictly defined areas and nurses who are GP-attached may have to travel a lot.

Coverage of services There are at least two countries that are not (yet) fully covered by community nursing services for the adult and elderly population: France and Germany.

For-profit versus non-profit All organizations taken into account in this study were non-profit. In all countries taken into account community nursing organizations are usually non-profit. In many countries, however, cost-containment measures include the introduction of competitive elements in the health care system. This may mean the advent of a for-profit sector, also in community nursing. This advent is feared by many.

The United States was the only country in this study with a substantial for-profit sector in community nursing (Table 10.7). A study by Shuster and Cloonan (1991) provides information on the differences in case management and patient populations between these two types of agencies. A comparison of the overall findings concerning case management revealed only marginal differences, though nurses working for for-profit agencies appeared to spend less time on direct care and more on indirect care activities. A bigger difference was found concerning patient populations. For-profit agencies had a higher percentage of Medicare patients and lower percentages of Medicaid, self-pay and indigent patients. The most striking difference, however, appears in the average number of visits per patient: 10 with for-profit agencies and 21 with non-profit agencies.

These are differences that should be carefully considered when countries start to introduce competitive elements into their health care systems.

Table 10.7
Relative number of for-profit community nursing agencies

	many	some	practically none
Belgium			x
Canada			x
Finland			x
France		x	
Germany		x	
Netherlands		x	
Norway			x
United Kingdom			x
United States	x		

Reimbursement There are two main principles according to which reimbursement can be made; fee for service and lump sums.

A. *Fee for service* There are various types of reimbursement on a fee for service basis. In the most simple type reimbursement is made in terms of a nomenclature. This nomenclature contains a list of activities and states the cost of these activities. This price can be reimbursed to the community nursing organization or to the patient. This system is part of the reimbursement system in France and Belgium.

Reimbursement can also take place based on the number of home visits. Here a distinction can be made between various types of home visits according to the type of care that is delivered during these visits. This is the case in Germany. In the USA reimbursement is usually based on the number of visits.

A third type of fee for service reimbursement is based on the number of days of care. This is part of the system in Belgium as far as heavily or moderately patients are concerned. The sum that is reimbursed varies with the level of dependency of the patient.

B. *Lump sums* The most simple form of this type of reimbursement prevails in England, Finland, Norway, the Netherlands and Canada (Ontario). In Finland and Norway the lump sums are paid to the local governments and are dependent on the number of inhabitants and prosperity of the local community. In England the sum is paid to the district health authorities. In Canada (Ontario) the provincial government pays to the local branches of the Victorian Order of Nurses. In the Netherlands the central government pays the regional cross associations.

In France a special form of the lump sum method exists, in addition to the nomenclature system. Here the organization is authorised by the sick funds to care for a fixed number of patients under the HAD and SAD schemes and gets reimbursed accordingly per patient.

Concerning reimbursement a number of recent developments are note-worthy. First the recent shift in Belgium to reimbursement per day of care, which varies between highly dependent and moderately dependent patients.

Second, a comparable development is taking place in France. In a recent government publication it is suggested that reimbursement for elderly care be made dependent on the level of dependency of the patient. According to Tophoven (1991), a similar change is being discussed in Germany too.

Co-payment Co-payments are quite common in all countries with respect to prescribed drugs and medical services. In most countries, however, community nursing services are free of charge (see Table 10.8).

All countries have co-payment for home help services, usually dependent on income of the recipient.

Table 10.8
Co-payment for community nursing in nine countries

	yes / no	if yes amount
Belgium	dependent on insurance	membership fee + cost dependent on insurance
Canada	no	--
UK	no	--
Finland	no	--
France	dependent on insurance	dependent on insurance
Germany	no	--
Netherlands	yes	membership fee yearly
Norway	no	--
USA	dependent on insurance	dependent on insurance

Maxima to the amount of care Funding bodies may state maxima to the amount of care that can be obtained. In Belgium, England, Finland and Norway no statutory limitations were reported.

In Canada there is entitlement to 3-4 visits per day for a limited period after which 1-2 visits per day is usually the maximum.

In France (Santé Service Charente) there is entitlement to 4 visits of 30 minutes per day by nurses and 2 visits (or 1.5 hour) a day by auxiliaries.

In Germany compulsorily insured persons are entitled to three visits per day

189

for four weeks for Behandlungspflege, beyond which special permission by the Health Insurance fund is necessary. For home help and Grundpflege there is a maximum of 25 visits a month.

In the Netherlands there is entitlement to 2.5 hours or 3 visits per day.

In the USA the maximum visits are dependent on the patient's insurance.

In most countries exceptions are made for care for terminally ill patients. This care is usually delivered by special organizations.

Types of community nurses and manpower

General Two main distinctions can be made between types of nurses:
- between levels of expertise
- between tasks: child health care and adult/elderly care.

In all countries there appeared to be at least two levels of expertise.

The Netherlands appeared to be the only country in which there were no separate types of nurses for child health care on the one hand and for adult-/elderly care on the other. In this country, community nurses work as generalists. However, in the near future most Dutch community nurses will also specialize in either mother and child care or adult/elderly care. In all other countries most nurses were assigned to either of these categories of care and very often had different training also.

Education The length of training of various types of nurses is shown in Table 10.9. Interpretation of this table is quite hazardous since no information is given about the various courses that can be taken by nurses to increase their knowledge. Secondly, no information is given on the length of previous training. The table only gives information about the most common types of nurse in the various countries and the minimal qualifications for each specific type of nurse.

In general the length of training for the first level of expertise varies between 3 and 5 years. The length of training for the lowest level of expertise varies between 1 and 3 years. In most countries there is a special training scheme for public health nursing. Special training for home nursing is less common and often takes place in courses instead of day schools. It must be noted, however that home nursing is becoming a more and more important part in the general nursing training programme in some countries. This was reported in Norway and Britain.

In the UK, Canada, USA, Germany, Finland, Belgium and the Netherlands the existence or introduction of university programmes on nursing science were reported.

Table 10.9
Basic training of various types of nurses in nine countries and
% of time spent on practical training

country	types of nurses	length of studies	% practical*
Belgium	social nurse	4 year	n.a.
	graduated nurse	3 year	62%
	brevetted nurse	3 year	n.a.
	hospital assistant nurse	2 year	n.a.
Canada	clinical nurse specialist	4 year university	n.a.
	public health nurse	4 year university	n.a.
	registered general nurse	2-3 year college	n.a.
	registered nurse assistant	1 year college	n.a.
Finland	specialist nurse	3,5-4,5 year	n.a.
situation	(among which public		
after 1987	health nurses)		
	practical nurses	1,5-2,5 year	n.a.
France	infirmière	3 year nursing school	51%
	aide soignante	1 year auxiliary school	n.a.
Germany	(Kinder)krankenschwester	3 year	65%
	Altenpfleger	3 year	46-55%
	Krankenpflegehilfe	1 year	69%
Netherlands	wijkverpleegkundige	4-5 year	39%
	wijkziekenverzorgende	3 year	n.a.
Norway	public health nurse	4 year	n.a.
	registered nurse	3 year	n.a.
	auxiliary	2 year	n.a.
UK	registered nurse	3 year	80%
	district nurse	4 year	n.a.
	public health nurse	4 year	n.a.
	enrolled nurse	2 year	n.a.
	auxiliary	varies	n.a.
USA	registered nurse	varies	n.a.
	licenced practical nurse	1 year	n.a.

*   (Source: information handout at the 'premier colloque infirmier d'Europe, Strassbourg 5-6-7 Fevrier, 1991 and Schnell, 1987)

n.a. = information not available

Manpower Though we tried to compute nurse:population ratios for various countries a cross national comparison is not legitimate. For many countries we only possessed organization-specific information, for other countries the information was quite old and for other countries the information was region-specific. Another obscuring factor was the division of tasks between various types of nurses. For example, a comparison between the Dutch wijkverpleeg-kundigen and the English district nurse is impossible since the Dutch wijkver-pleegkundige also provides child health care, while in England this is left to another type of nurse. Adding the two types of nurses in England and conse-quently comparing them with the Dutch nurses is not possible since tasks performed by the Dutch nurses are sometimes provided by practical nurses in England. Furthermore, in many countries there is a large category of occu-pational nurses and independent nurses. In short: there are too many divisions of tasks among too many types of nurses in too many countries to draw general conclusions about nurse: population ratios.

However hazardous, it was still considered useful to look at the way in which levels of expertise relate to each other. Table 10.10 gives the ratios between levels of expertise in the seven countries. Much is dependent on the definition of first and lower levels in each country and the figures should be considered with much caution, but it is legitimate to state that Belgium and France have a high number of second level nurses compared to other countries. It has to be noted, however, that there is no difference in tasks between graduate and brevetted nurses in Belgium.

Table 10.10
Ratio between levels of expertise in seven countries

Belgium (White-Yellow Cross, liberales excluded)
graduated nurse : brevetted : hospital assistant nurse   1 : 1.5 : 0.2
Finland
public health : registered nurses : practical nurses   1 : 0.3 : 0.3
France (SAD-services in 1984)
Infirmières + liberales : aides soignantes   1 : 1
Germany
Krankenschwester : Altenpflegerin : Krankenpflegehelferin   1 : 0.2 : 0.1
Netherlands
wijkverpleegkundige : wijkziekenverzorgende   1 : 0.3
Norway
Nurses : auxiliaries   1 : 0.4
United Kingdom (District Nursing)
Registered nurses : enroled nurses   1 : 0.5

Patient populations

The most important distinction that can be made in patient populations is that between adults/elderly and children. It could be seen in all countries that the age groups between 10 and 60 form only a small part of the patient population. In both the Scandinavian countries, England and the Netherlands there is one organization for both types of care. The Netherlands is the only country in which children and adults are cared for by the same nurse though this method of working is currently being re-introduced in Finland. For all organizations that specialize in adult care 70 to 90% of the patients were above 65 years of age. In countries for which this information was available, the largest part of the people cared for consisted of women.

Worth mentioning here is the very high percentage (27%) of the total population that had had contact with a public health nurse in Finland. In countries for which this information was available, it was always below 10%. This may be an indication that nurses in Finland have tasks that are reserved for physicians in other countries.

Types of care

All countries taken into account deliver a comprehensive range of care for the elderly population.

In all countries nurses spend most of their time on home visits. Estimates of the percentage of the total working time spent on home visits varied between 60 and 90%. The estimates for administrative activities varied between 20 and 30%.

In some countries the type of reimbursement varies according to the type of care that is delivered. On the other hand, the types of care that are delivered are also dependent on the reimbursement system. Compared with the Netherlands, for instance, in Belgium very little time is spent on preventive activities because these activities are not represented in the 'nomenclature' on the basis of reimbursement is made.

Stages in Nursing

The distribution of the total number of patients over various sources of referral can be considered an indication for the level of independence of nurses in organizations and their need for skills that are necessary in judging the patient situation. It is assumed that these skills are more necessary where there is a larger percentage of self-referring patients not referred by a GP.

In addition, the proportion of hospital referrals can be considered as an indication for the quality of the relations between hospital and community nursing organizations (see also next section). The figures are presented in

Table 10.11.

The table shows large differences between the countries. The 99% referral by 'other' in Canada is due to the existence of a hospital based co-ordinator of home care who does not only refer from hospitals but also from home. The Belgian White-Yellow Cross definitely has the highest proportion of self-referrals, and England the lowest. It has to be noted, however, that most of the self-initiators in Belgium already have a prescription from a GP.

Table 10.11
Initiators of first contact with community nursing organizations
in nine countries

	patient self or family	GP	hospital or nursing-home	other
Belgium White Yellow Cross	80%	5%	15%	--
Canada(VON Ontario)	--	--	--	99% (co-ordinator)
England (District Nursing)	5%	40%	40%	15% (home help, other carers)
Finland (all public health nurses)	n o d a t a a v a i l a b l e			
France HAD	37%	10%	52%	1%
SAD (Santé Service Charente)	55%	14%	11%	18% (HAD)
Germany	n o d a t a a v a i l a b l e			
Netherlands	47%	17%	33%	9%
Norway	n o d a t a a v a i l a b l e			
USA (Visiting nurse service New York)	16%	5%	79%	--

Assessment of the patient's need is usually done by community nurses with the first level of expertise. Assessment of *medical need*, however, is a physician's task in all countries. In some countries a physician's prescription is needed for *all types of care* necessary for reimbursement (France, Germany, and the United States). In Belgium this is only true with the exception of hygienic care.

The decision as to which nurse is going to deliver the care is in most countries determined by where the patient lives, since in most countries nurses are assigned to a specific geographic area.

Evaluation is usually not formalized and takes often place on an ad-hoc basis. In France, Germany and the USA the patient's need should be periodically re-assessed by a physician.

Relations with general practitioners, home help services and hospitals

All community nursing organizations in all countries maintain relations with home help services, general practitioners and hospitals. In most countries the general practitioners are the ones with whom most contact takes place. Contact with home help services and hospitals is usually less frequent. In view of the existence of special personnel to maintain relations with other care providers, this is a matter of concern in many countries.

For almost all medical prescriptions the nurse is dependent on the general practitioner or other physician. However, limited nurse prescribing was reported to be discussed in the United Kingdom and the Netherlands and to be existing in the United States (mainly by university trained nurse practitioners). It was reported that in France and Germany and the USA hygienic care has to be prescribed by a doctor too.

The number of general practitioners with whom a nurse has to deal varies in all countries according to degree of urbanization. England and Finland are the only countries with GP-attached nurses.

In all countries there are organizations that offer community nursing as well as home help care, but this is not true for all organizations. In organizations where this is not the case, co-operation and co-ordination takes usually place on an ad-hoc basis.

There seems to be a trend in many countries to integrate home help services and community nursing services one way or another.

Contacts with hospital personnel usually take place on an ad-hoc basis also. In some countries, however, there are nurses who are especially assigned to maintaining relations between hospitals and community nursing organizations. Sometimes these nurses are hospital based, sometimes they are community based.

Problems

Underperformance In all countries respondents to the questionnaire were asked to indicate what community nursing tasks they considered underperformed.

Not surprisingly, most of these underperformed tasks are connected with the elderly population. Most frequently mentioned were psychosocial activities and stimulation of care by friends, family and relatives. The connection between these two is obvious: more informal care means less work for nurses and consequently more time for psychosocial activities. Another reason for the need for more psychosocial activities (and informal care) is of course the shortage of community nurses in general. In some countries this shortage is only threatening, in others it is already a very real problem.

In respect of encouragement of informal care, Germany is noteworthy. In Germany patients can organize the care themselves and receive 400 DM per month to do this. This applies only to 'Grundpflege' and home help services. In this country informal carers who have taken care of a patient for twelve months can take a holiday and receive a sum of money to organize the care during this holiday. Germany seems to be the only country in which there are financial incentives for informal carers.

Personnel shortages All countries reported a (threatening) shortage of community nurses. Cut-and-dried solutions to this problem were found nowhere.

In some countries it was reported that hospital nurses were paid better than community nurses and that would help equal payment.

Also, an increasing number of part-timers was reported to be a reason for shortages of personnel, as well as the fact that nurses stay in the profession only a short time.

Delegating less complicated tasks to lower staff was suggested in England. In most countries, however, (in England also) there is only a very small quantity of lower level staff available. The two countries with a relatively large proportion of second level personnel are Belgium and France. In Belgium, however, there is no difference in tasks between the two levels (brevetted nurses and graduate nurses).

Specialist versus generalist There are two ways in which this problem can be looked at.
1   Should there be a division between (preventive) child health care and (curative) elderly care?
The Netherlands, England and Finland are the three countries in which this is a problematic issue.

The Netherlands is the only country in which the same nurse takes care of the child health care as well as the elderly care. This truly all-round method of working is under discussion and it is foreseen by many that a division between the two types of care will take place in the near future.

On the other hand there is Finland. After several years of experience with the specialist approach, people in Finland are considering the re-introduction of the generalist nurse. This is expected to increase the involvement of nurses in the community and vice-versa. In sparsely populated areas in particular the specialist method of working involved a lot of travelling for nurses.

In England the existing division between preventive care and curative care causes problems. Care for healthy elderly is considered to be a task for health visitors and care for the sick elderly is considered to be a task for district nurses. Some people question the efficiency of this division. Communication between the two types of nurses is often difficult because they work in separate teams.

England is the only country in which difficulties in the existing division of curative and preventive tasks were reported. In all other countries this does not seem a major problem.

2   Should there be a division of tasks within curative elderly care?
In all countries except the Netherlands (and to some extent Finland) there are separate nurses for preventive child health care and curative elderly care and few problems are reported concerning this division. This, however, does not mean that there is no need for specialists within curative elderly care. In many countries there is a limited number of specialist nurses whose main task it usually is to advise colleagues.

Levels of expertise and home helps The division of tasks between different levels nurses seems to be a problem in some countries.

From England assigning less esoteric care to lower levels of staff was suggested as a solution to personnel shortages. The problem, however, is that there are relatively few lower level nursing staff in almost all countries.

The division of tasks between nurses and home helps was reported to be a problem in only a few countries.

Community nursing and general practitioner In all countries nurses are dependent on prescriptions by physicians for *medical interventions*, except for the nurse practitioners in the US. In some countries, however, this applies to *all activities* (France, Germany and the US). This is sometimes considered to be a problem because it erodes the autonomy of the nurses.

In England most nurses are GP-attached and this involves a good deal of travel relatively speaking.

Hospital and community nursing In some countries communications between community nursing and hospital are a matter of concern. In some countries there are liaison nurses, who usually work in hospitals.

Funding In some countries the method of funding causes problems. In Belgium, for instance, the nomenclature does not include preventive and psychosocial activities. Regional differences in reimbursement of home care were reported from France. In France and Germany it was considered undesirable that home help and community nursing care be funded differently. A general lack of resources for community nursing was reported from most countries.

References

OECD (1988), *Ageing populations; the social policy implications*, Organization for economic co-operation and development, Paris.

Shuster, G.F. and P.A. Cloonan (1991), 'Home Health Nursing Care: A comparison of not-for-profit and for-profit agencies', *Home Health Care Services Review Quarterly*, 12, 1.

Statistical Yearbook of Norway 1990 (1990), Statistisk Sentralbyrå, Oslo-Kongsvingen.

Tophoven, L. (1991), *Die Absicherung des Pflegerisikos aussichte der GKV*, In: Arbeit und Sozialpolitik, 3-4.

Appendix 1

List of respondents and reviewers

Mrs. R. Sullivan, RN, M.H.Sc.
Regional Director Public Health Nursing
P.O.Box 8700
Forest Road
St. John's
NEW FOUNDLAND A1B4G6 CANADA

Mrs. J. Goeppinger M.A. Ph.D.
Prof. of Nursing and Area Chair
Community Health Nursing
School of Nursing University of Michigan
400 N. Ingalls
ANN ARBOR MICHIGAN 48109 USA

Mrs. D.M. Pringle RN, Ph.D.
Dean Faculty of Nursing
University of Toronto
50 St. Georgestreet
TORONTO ONTARIO M5S1A1 CANADA

Mrs. K. Lonergan
Director of Business Development
Visiting Nurse Services of New York
350 Fith Avenue, Suite 441
NEW YORK, NY 10118 USA

Mr. H. van Loon, general manager
Nationale Federatie Wit-Gele Kruis
Ad. Lacomblélaan 69
1040 BRUSSELS Belgium

Mrs. K. Buhler-Wilkerson
University of Pennsylvania
School of Nursing
420 Service Drive
PHILADELPHIA PA 19104-6096 USA

Mr. T. Butterworth, professor
Department of Nursing
New Medical School Stopford
Oxford Road
MANCHESTER 13 9PT UK

Mr. B. Pateman
Department of Nursing
New Medical School Stopford
Oxford Road
MANCHESTER 13 9PT UK

Mrs. J. Merrell
Department of Nursing
New Medical School Stopford
Oxford Road
MANCHESTER 13 9PT UK

Mrs. C. Niclausse, délégué général
Centre d'animation pour soins et services
aux personne agées (C.A.S.S.P.A.)
35 Boulevard Jeanne d'Arc
02200 SOISSONS France

Mrs. L.M. Shortridge
Professor and associate dean
Lienhard School of Nursing
Lienhard Hall 304
861 Bedford Road
Pleasantville, NY 10570 USA

Mr. L. Geys, responsable departement nursing
Nationale Federatie Wit-Gele Kruis
Ad. Lacomblélaan 69-71
0040 BRUSSEL Belgium

Mrs. B. Ellefsen, assistant professor
Institutt for Sykepleievitenskap
Universitetet i Oslo
Postboks 1120 - Blindern
0317 OSLO 3 Norway

Mrs. M. Schwertl-Staubach, directeur
German Nurses' Association
Arndstrasse 15
D-6000 FRANKFURT AM MAIN 1 BRD

Mrs. M. Rustad, International Secretary
Norwegian Nurses Association
PO Box 2633 - St. Hanshaugen
0131 OSLO 1 Norway

Mrs. Judith Harris, RN, M.P.H.
Visiting Nurse Association
Greater Philadelphia
One Winding Drive
PHILADELPHIA, PA 19131-2992 USA

Mrs. P. Koponen, RN, M.Sc.
University of Tampere
Department of Public Health
P.O.Box 607
SF - 33101 TAMPERE Finland

Mr. J. Korporal, Prof. Dr.
Fachhochschule für Sozialarbeit und Sozialpädagogik
Karl-Chrader-Strasse 6
1000 BERLIN 10 Germany

Mr. L. Vandenberghe
Dienst Kind en Gezin
Hallepoortlaan 27
1060 BRUSSEL Belgium

Mr. D. Demeester, Head Community Nursing
Solidariteit voor het Gezin
Tentoonstellingsstraat 72
9000 GENT Belgium

Mr. F. Brandt, Dipl.Soz.
Institut für Sozialforschung und Sozialwirtschaft
Trillerweg 68
6600 SAARBRÜCKEN Germany

Mr. Rudolf Schweikart
Institut für Sozialforschung
und Sozialwirtschaft
Trillerweg 68
6600 SAARBRÜCKEN Germany

Mr. M. Schneider
BASYS GmbH
Reisinger Strasse 25
8900 AUGSBURG Germany

Mrs. Crinque
Association Medico-Sociale
Anne Morgan (A.M.S.A.M.)
31 rue Anne Morgan
02200 SOISSONS France

Docteur Lenquette
A.N.P.S.
B.P. 10
02700 TERGNIER France

Mrs. M. Gabanyi, M.A.
BASYS GmbH
Reisinger Strasse 25
8900 AUGSBURG Germany

Mrs. B.T. Dahlgren, assistant director
Professional Nursing Department
Norwegian Nurses Association
PO Box 2633 - St. Hanshaugen
0121 OSLO 1 Norway

Mrs. Gorski
Santé Service Charente
62-64 rue Saint-Roch
16006 ANGOULEME CEDEX   France

Appendix 2

List of organizations visited

DIDSBURY CLINIC
Mrs M. Graham / Mrs J. Saunders
828 Wilmslow Road
DIDSBURY England

CHORLTON HEALTH CENTRE
Mrs J. Canham / Mrs. C. Leather
1 Nicolas Road
MANCHESTER England

ZENTRALE AMBULANTE KRANKENPFLEGE
Frau Oldorf
Hammarskjöldring 75
6000 FRANKFURT 50 Germany

HÄUSLICHE KRANKENPFLEGEDIENST
Hr J. Limbach
Gossenburg 9
WUPPERTAL Germany

Association Médico Sociale Anne Morgan
Mme Crinque
31 Rue Anne Morgan
02200 SOISSONS FRANCE

Santé Service Charente
Mme Gorski
62 Rue Saint-Roch
16014 ANGOULEME CEDEX FRANCE

PHOJANAHON NEUVOLA
Mrs V. Pennanen
Pohjanaho 2
40520 JYVÄSKYLÄ Finland

KIIKANMÄEN NEUVOLA
Mrs M. Kilpeläinen
Sairaalantie
35100 ORIVESI Finland

Appendix 3

The population responsibility project
(adapted from Liukko et al. 1990)

The project is a practical experiment to support the local implementation of the principle of population responsibility. It is a management project where local independency is supported and the central administration's role is more supportive than directive.

The project is divided into four subprojects:
1 The general practitioner project. The most important aspect of this project is that a GP is assigned to a small geographical area. Secondly, an experiment is being carried out with a new system of reimbursement (see section 4.1.2). The other subprojects stem from the general practitioner project.
2 The public health nurse project. Identical geographical boundaries with general practitioners.
3 Occupational health care project will study the role of occupational health care in primary care.
4 The social services and primary care collaboration project will study teamwork between health and social services.

Most interesting for our purposes is the public health nurse project. Three models are studied:
1 The comprehensive model (15% of the nurses in the study)
   The public health nurse will deliver all or almost all the different services needed by the small population.
2 The semi-comprehensive model (35% of the nurses in the study)
   The public health nurse will deliver 3-4 different kinds of services needed by the population. The ambulatory medical care is delivered

207

according to a small area list of 1500 - 2000 citizens. For the rest of the services two to four of these small areas are united and in this larger area are public health nurse is responsible for the maternal care, another for the child care etc.

3   The specialised model (50% of the nurses in the study)
The general practitioner or the public health nurse delivers one service to the population e.g. maternal or child care.

An important part of the project is to describe the population of the health centres participating in the project.
Secondly the structure of the use of health services will be studied. These health services also include other than those delivered by health centres.
The aim is to make out what works best where and with what population.

Data are gathered from about 10 health centres through:
-    interviewing the population
-    questionnaire for patients
-    registration of patient contacts
-    questionnaire for personnel
-    group interviews with personnel and observing teamwork
-    comparing local statistics.

Appendix 4

Future developments in the organization of community nursing in England
(adapted from: North West Thames Regional Health Authority. Nursing in
the Community, report of the working group, 1991)

The report of the working group Nursing in the Community mentions five
models for the organization and management of the nursing services in the
community. It is for the managers and practitioners at local level to decide
whether individual models or a combination of two or more best meets the
local needs.

The models differ particularly in the degree of GP participation and in the
degree of integration between various types of care.

A The 'Stand Alone' Community Trust or DMU

Under this model the community (nursing) unit would manage all
community health services and offer (sell) them to local GPs, units
providing secondary care, local authorities, voluntary agencies and the
independent sector.

B Locality Management/ Neighbourhood Nursing Model

Under this model, mixed teams of community staff would be managed in
localities arranged either in geographicl patches or around consortia of GP
practices of health centers under the overall control of the community unit.

C Expanded FHSA Model

Under this model the Family Health Service Authority would assume
responsibility for the provision of community services under an agency
arrangement with the District Health Authority.

D Vertical Integration or Outreach Model

This model could take a variety of forms such as a combined acute/
community unit; an acute unit; unit providing secondary care with
community outreach; or a community unit with acute outreach.

E Primary Health Care Team (PHCT) - GP managed

Under this model, community services would be brought under the control and management of general practice.